The ECG Manual

Marc Gertsch

The ECG Manual

An Evidence-Based Approach

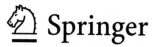 Springer

Marc Gertsch, MD
Department of Cardiology
University Clinic Inselspital
Bern
Switzerland

ISBN 978-1-84800-170-1   e-ISBN 978-1-84800-171-8
DOI 10.1007/978-1-84800-171-8

British Library Cataloguing in Publication Data

Gertsch, Marc
    The ECG manual: an evidence-based approach
    1. Electrocardiography   2. Evidence-based medicine
    I. Title
    616.1'207547

Library of Congress Control Number: 2008923737

Printed on acid-free paper

9 8 7 6 5 4 3 2 1

springer.com

Foreword

Marc Gertsch is a true expert in the ECG and its analysis. In this small book, intended for medical students, house-staff, residents, and coronary care/intensive therapy unit nurses, the author eliminates much of the ritual explanation of the derivation of the electrocardiogram and, instead, provides a pragmatic and practical approach to its interpretation. The book explores important principles of electrocardiology and importantly electrocardiographic traces are consistently related to clinical scenarios and real-life cases.

The art of ECG interpretation is often shrouded in mystique but an important principle that Professor Gertsch uses throughout this book is to base his explanation of the ECG findings on evidence from the literature. In this way the "secret" of the ECG is thoroughly exposed and it becomes possible to use the technique to reach accurate and practical diagnoses.

These days many physicians rely on the automatic analysis of an ECG by a computer chip on board the ECG recording machine. It has even been suggested that such "diagnosis" is now so correct that it might be possible not print the tracing itself. This would reduce the physician's familiarity and understanding of the ECG still further. As with the modern echocardiogram, we may expect to see only the reports of studies, and it will be left to our memories to relate the report to similar examples of findings seen in the past. Professor Gertsch's book dispels this notion by explaining how the simple way in which an ECG may be interpreted and the essential aspect of making that interpretation within a clinical context, something that no ECG machine yet attempts to do!

Above all Marc Gertsch is a teacher, and a demanding teacher at that. He expects his students to learn and with this book he has provided the material for study. It is a pleasure and an education to read.

A. John Camm
Professor Clinical Cardiology
St George's University of London
UK

Preface

This book is designed for medical students and colleagues (including general practitioners, internists, and cardiologists) who need a short, practical book to help them correctly interpret more than 90% of all ECGs they see on a daily basis. Although this is a particularly ambitious goal for such a compact ECG book, important theoretic basics, as well as ventricular and atrial *vectors*, are included.

The knowledge needed to correctly identify diagnostic ECG features, including arrhythmias, requires extensive experience obtained over many years. Why then an "evidence-based" book? Because the cardiologist must be experienced in all fields of cardiology: in the ambulatory section using Echo/Doppler, ambulatory, and exercise ECGs; at the emergency station; and in the coronary care unit. The interventional cardiologist, who has performed thousands of heart catheterizations, coronary angiographies, and pacemaker implantations, and has moved beyond field into invasive electrophysiology, has a *very critical* attitude toward ECGs. Such cardiologists always respect the *limits* of ECGs when compared with other approaches, such as echocardiographic or coronary angiographic findings.

Another argument for an "evidence-based" book is that I read or re-read more than 2000 citations, of which approximately 650 have been included in this book. The evidence was improved by adding detailed descriptions of the coronary artery and left ventricular angiographic findings for every of the thirty ECG patterns of myocardial infarction, as well as by case reports/short stories of predominantly spectacular cases.

Designed to sit alongside my earlier publication, *The ECG: A Two-Step Approach to Diagnosis*, references to that book are given if the details cannot be found in any other ECG book (e.g., a long list of the etiology of electrolyte disturbances, the differentiation of myocardial infarction stages based on four principally different nomenclatures, and the ECG documentation of *all* possible false limb lead poling in electric left and vertical hearts).

It remains to thank my young academic collaborator Christoph Obrecht for extensive logistic help and meticulous corrections, to my excellent scientific designer Willy Hess, to Sandra Fabiani, Senior Editor at Springer Heidelberg with whom all this began, to Barbara Chernow from Chernow Editorial Services Inc., New York, and to Grant Weston, Senior Editor at Springer London for constructive and pleasant collaboration.

Marc Gertsch, MD
June 2008

Contents

Abbreviations

The following abbreviations are used regularly throughout the text:

AAI pacing   Atrial inhibited atrial pacing
ACE   Angiotensin-converting enzyme
acPE   Acute pulmonary embolism
AF   Atrial fibrillation
AJT   Automatic junctional tachycardia
AMI   Acute myocardial infarction
AP or acP   Action potential
APB   Atrial premature beat
$\mathring{A}QRS_F$ Mean QRS axis in the frontal plane
ASD   Atrial septal defect
AV   Atrioventricular
AVR   Aortic valve replacement
AVNRT   Atrioventricular nodal reentrant tachycardia

BVH   Biventricular hypertrophy

CABG   Coronary artery bypass graft
CAD   Coronary artery disease
CHD   Coronary heart disease
CK = CPK   Creatine kinase
CK-MB   Myocardial-bound creatine kinase
COPD   Chronic obstructive pulmonary disease
Coro   Coronary angiogram/coronary angiography. (In most cases, "coro" also includes left ventricular angiography/angiogram.)
CPK   Creatine phosphokinase
CPR   Cardiopulmonary resuscitation
CT   Computed tomography
CX   Circumflexa (circumflex branch of the left coronary artery)

DC   Direct current
DD   Differential diagnosis

DDD	Dual-chamber dual-inhibited (pacing)
DDD(R)	Dual-chamber dual-inhibited rate responsive (pacing)
ECG	Electrocardiogram
Echo	Echocardiogram/echocardiography (in most cases color Doppler is integrated)
EF	Ejection fraction (in most cases of the left ventricle)
EPI/EPS	Electrophysiologic investigation/study
HOCM	Hypertrophic obstructive cardiomyopathy
Htx	Xeno-transplantation of the heart
ICD	Implantable cardioverter defibrillator
INR	International normalized ratio (for oral anticoagulation)
LA	Left atrium/left atrial
LAD	Left anterior descending coronary artery = left anterior descending branch of the left coronary artery
LAD	Left axis deviation ($\overset{\circ}{A}QRS_F < -30°$)
LAFB	Left anterior fascicular block (= left anterior "hemiblock")
LBBB	(Complete) left bundle-branch block
LCA	Left coronary artery
LPFB	Left posterior fascicular block (= left posterior "hemiblock")
LV	Left ventricle/left ventricular
LVH	Left ventricular hypertrophy
MET	Metabolic equivalents
MET	Maximal exercise test
MI	Myocardial infarction
MAS attack	Morgagni-Adams-Stokes attack
MRI	Magnetic resonance imaging
NSAID	Nonsteroidal antiinflammatory drug
PA	Pulmonary artery
PE	Pulmonary embolism
PET	Positron emission tomography
PJRT	Permanent junctional reciprocating tachycardia
PTCA	Percutaneous coronary transluminal angioplasty
RA	Right atrium/right atrial
RBBB	(Complete) right bundle-branch block
RCA	Right coronary artery
RV	Right ventricle/right ventricular
RVD	Right ventricular dysplasia
RVOT	Right ventricular outflow tract

SA	Sinoatrial
SACT	Sinoatrial conduction time
SN	Sinus node
SNRT	Sinus node recovery time
SPECT	Single photon emission computed tomography
SR	Sinus rhythm
SVPB	Supraventricular premature beat
SVT	Supraventricular tachycardia
SVTab	Supraventricular tachycardia with aberration
VPB	Ventricular premature beat
VSD	Ventricular septal defect
VT	Ventricular tachycardia
VVI	One-chamber ventricular (pacemaker)
VVI(R)	Ventricular inhibited ventricular rate-responsive (pacing)
WPW syndrome	Wolff-Parkinson-White syndrome

Chapter 1
Some Theoretic Aspects

Because every physician, and even more so, every student in medicine, is aware of the important theoretic basics of Electrocardiology [as anatomy and the impulse conduction system, correlation between ion flows and the intracellular action potential (AP) of a single myocardial working cell, lead systems, and the nomenclature of the heart cycle], repetition in this short *ECG Manual* is renounced. Only some lesser-known basics are provided. Moreover, the reader will find a section about the determination of the frontal QRS axis ($\mathring{A}QRS_F$).

Atrial vectors are discussed in Chapter 3, "**The Normal Electrocardiogram and Its (Normal) Variants**." The ventricular vectors, however, are discussed in this chapter, and a simplified scheme of the left ventricular vectors is provided that is especially useful in understanding bundle-branch blocks and the fact that the human electrocardiogram (ECG) generally represents a "levogram."

Differences Among Heart Cells

In Figure 1.1a–c, the main differences of AP among (a) a working cell, (b) a conduction cell, and (c) a sinus node cell are demonstrated. In working fibers, phase 4 of the AP remains stable and isoelectric, respectively (Figure 1.1a). In contrast, conduction fibers have a slow depolarization during phase 4, called *slow spontaneous phase 4 (diastolic) depolarization*. This also represents an inherent characteristic of a pacemaker cell and explains the potential capacity of a conduction cell to act as pacemaker cell. If the cell is not depolarized by an electrical stimulus before reaching the threshold at the level of approximately −70 mV, it spontaneously depolarizes (Figure 1.1b). This fact is important for the understanding of arrhythmia, e.g., in premature and escape beats and rhythms.

A ventricular premature beat is generated by a diseased Purkinje cell (or a group of fibers) that shows a faster "spontaneous phase 4 depolarization" than the sinus node. Thus, the premature beat falls in too early (as the term describes it), disturbing the normal rhythm.

In contrast, an escape beat falls in too late, visually. For example, in the case of complete infrahisian atrioventricular block, asystole would occur, without a

M. Gertsch, *The ECG Manual: An Evidence-Based Approach*,
© Springer-Verlag London Limited 2009

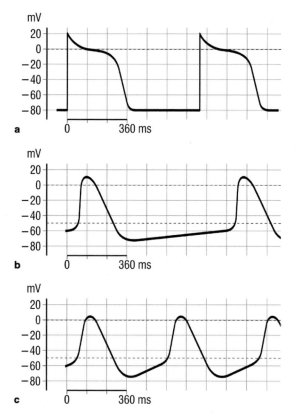

Figure 1.1 a. Action potential (AP) of a single working heart muscle cell. **b.** AP of a single conduction cell. **c.** AP of a single sinus node cell

ventricular escape beat (or rhythm). Because no electric stimulus reaches the Purkinje fibers, their "spontaneous phase 4 depolarization potential" reaches the threshold and produces an AP, an ordinary depolarization. The Purkinje fibers substitute the absent rhythm in a beneficial manner, at a lower rate.

As mentioned, the shape of the AP between conduction cells and pacemaker cells is not principally different. However, a relatively fast "slow spontaneous phase 4 depolarization," associated with a short AP (both resulting in a relative high rate), allows the pacemaker fibers to depolarize first. In normal conditions, the fibers of the sinus node have the shortest AP, thus dominating the heart rhythm (Figure 1.1c).

Ventricular Vectors and Their Simplification

A vector is a theoretic model for an electric force. The different types are P vectors, QRS vectors, ST vectors, and T vectors. The concept of vectors, especially of the QRS vectors, with their amplitude and their directions in all three dimensions, is of great importance for understanding the scalar ECG, in normal and some pathologic conditions (such as bundle-branch blocks, fascicular blocks, left and right ventricular hypertrophy, and myocardial infarction).

Simplified QRS Vectors

The instantaneous vectorial interpretation, described here and later presented in a simplified manner, also considerably facilitates memorization of important ECG patterns (Figure 1.2). In normal conditions [and pathologic conditions, with the exclusion of left bundle-branch block (LBBB) and corrected transposition of the great arteries], ventricular excitation begins in the middle part of the interventricular septum on the left side and spreads out throughout the septum, from left to right. This first QRS vector (or septal vector), vector 1, lasts approximately 15 ms, is generally directed to the right, anteriorly and slightly downward, and corresponds to the small Q wave in leads I and V_5/V_6. In other leads (for instance in V_1/V_2), the same vector leads to a small R wave, because of projection.

Afterward, the apical part of the left ventricle is depolarized, followed by the excitation of the main portions of the left (and right) ventricle. The great second QRS vector, vector 2, lasts approximately 60 ms, is generally directed to the left, inferiorly and mostly slightly posteriorly, and corresponds to the tall R waves in leads I and V_5/V_6 and the deep S waves in V_2/V_3. The great left ventricular main vector completely swallows the small simultaneous right ventricular, vector 2a, produced by the depolarization of the right ventricle, with its muscle mass 15 times

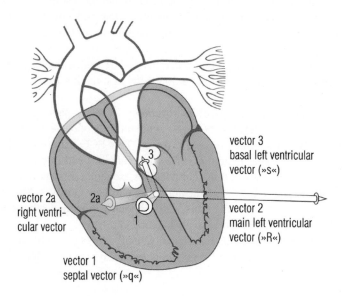

vector 3
basal left ventricular
vector (»s«)

vector 2a
right ventri-
cular vector

vector 2
main left ventricular
vector (»R«)

vector 1
septal vector (»q«)

Figure 1.2 Simplified QRS vectors

smaller than the left ventricle muscle mass. In regard to ventricular depolarization (and repolarization), the human ECG represents a "levogram." Right ventricular activation is only visible in the ECG in conditions that increase the right ventricle vector (in right ventricular hypertrophy) or delay right ventricle excitation [in right bundle-branch block (RBBB)].

The remaining small upper ventricular parts (of the high lateral wall of the left and right ventricle and the upper part of the septum) are excited last. The third small QRS vector, vector 3, lasts approximately 15 ms, points generally superiorly, to the right and posteriorly and leads in the ECG to the small S wave in lead I/V_6 and to the last part of the S wave in lead V_2/V_3.

The QRS configuration in an ECG lead depends on the variations of the frontal QRS axis (the variations in the horizontal plane are of minor degree), and on the projection of the three above-mentioned ventricular vectors on the different ECG leads in the frontal and horizontal plane. A QRS complex may also be an RS complex, a QS complex, or a simple R wave, and so on.

ST and T Alterations in the Different Stages of Ischemia

The nomenclature of the different grades of ischemia is shown in Figure 1.3. The expressions for ischemia used below represent electrocardiographic terms, and include the different grades of hypoxia of (mostly left) ventricular myocardium.

The slightest grade of ischemia manifests as high and peaked T waves and is called *subendocardial ischemia*. It has the same morphologic alteration found in moderate hyperkalemia. A higher grade of ischemia leads to the pattern of symmetric negative T waves. The term *subepicardial ischemia* is sometimes used. This same alteration is found in many conditions other than ischemia (see Chapter 17, "Alterations of Repolarization"). An even higher grade of ischemia leads to depression of the ST segment and is called *subendocardial lesion*. This alteration is also rather nonspecific and is seen in conditions such as left ventricular hypertrophy and in patients receiving digitalis. ST depression is the best marker for ischemia during exercise.

These three grades of ischemia are reversible in many patients. The highest grade leads to extensive elevation of the ST segment (monophasic deformation) and is called *transmural lesion* or *transmural injury*. This ECG pattern is only reversible in the case of vasospastic angina (Prinzmetal angina) and in other rare conditions. In approximately 99% of transmural lesions, ischemia persists and myocardial infarction (necrosis) develops, with the appearance of new Q waves. Minor degrees of ST elevation are seen in pericarditis, early repolarization, and other conditions, all in the absence of true ischemia (see Chapter 17).

It is important to mention that, theoretically, in all grades of electrocardiographic ischemia, the grade is highest in the subendocardial layers of the (left) ventricular myocardium.

Figure 1.3 T and ST alterations
in the different stages of ischemia

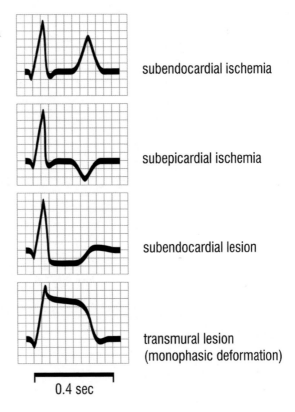

subendocardial ischemia

subepicardial ischemia

subendocardial lesion

transmural lesion
(monophasic deformation)

0.4 sec

Determination of the Mean Frontal QRS Axis

The triangle of Einthoven, shown in Figure 1.4 (in Figure 1.5 integrated in the circle of Cabrera), is the basis for the calculation of ÅQRS_F. Einthoven's triangle and Cabrera's circle represent a reasonable arbitrarily determined construction of a system of frontal leads and of degrees, subdivided in positive and negative degrees, where the cardiac vectors, especially the direction of the ÅQRS_F complex, can be placed.

In the German literature, the following inexact nomenclature is frequently used:

ÅQRS_F more positive than +120° = Überdrehte (QRS) Rechtslage
ÅQRS_F between +120° and +90° = Rechtslage
ÅQRS_F between +90° and +60° = Steillage
ÅQRS_F between +60° and +30° = Mittellage *or* Indifferenzlage
ÅQRS_F between +30° and −30° = Linkslage
ÅQRS_F less than −30° (more negative than −30°) = Überdrehte Linkslage

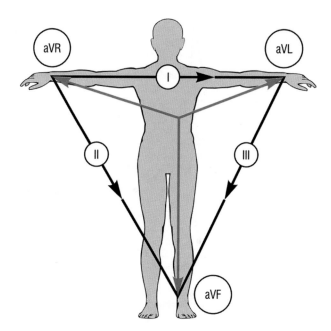

Figure 1.4 Einthoven's triangle

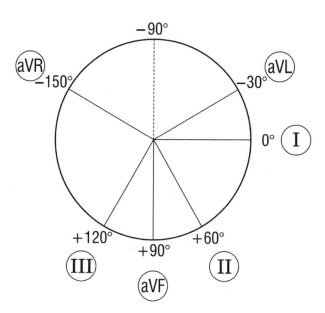

Figure 1.5 Cabrera's circle

In the English literature, only left axis deviation (more negative than −30°; this means between −30° and ±150°) and right axis deviation (more positive than +120°; this means between +120° and ±150°) are clearly defined. A vertical electric frontal QRS axis is approximately +90°, and a left frontal QRS approximately 0°.

In any case, it is more exact to calculate the $\mathring{A}QRS_F$ with a precision of approximately ±10°. This can be performed within several seconds, after some practice. It is important to mention that we always consider the *plane* of the positive and negative portions of QRS and *not* the amplitude.

Examples

Example 1 (Figure 1.6a)
The QRS in lead aVF is isoelectric. This means that the $\mathring{A}QRS_F$ is perpendicular (at an angle of 90°) to aVF. Therefore, $\mathring{A}QRS_F$ is +90° or −90°. Lead I shows a positive QRS, so $\mathring{A}QRS_F$ is 0°. Looking for an overall isoelectric QRS is the fastest method for determining $\mathring{A}QRS_F$.

Example 2 (Figure 1.6b)
In lead I, the QRS is slightly more positive than negative, in aVL, the QRS is a bit more negative than positive, and leads II and aVF show almost the same QRS configuration. $\mathring{A}QRS_F$ is calculated at approximately +80°.

Example 3 (Figure 1.6c)
QRS in I is a bit more negative than positive, but significantly more negative in aVL. The QRS is more positive than negative in II and aVF, but almost purely positive in III and nearly isoelectric in aVR. $\mathring{A}QRS_F$ is approximately +120°.

Example 4 (Figure 1.6d)
QRS is more positive in III and aVF than in II, more negative than positive in I, completely negative in aVL, and only slightly positive in aVR. $\mathring{A}QRS_F$ is approximately +110°.

In calculating the $\mathring{A}QRS_F$ in the presence of complete RBBB, the mean frontal left ventricular QRS vector is always. The right ventricular mean frontal QRS vector does not (or at best by some degrees) influence the $\mathring{A}QRS_F$ except in the presence of considerable right ventricle hypertrophy or in the presence of RBBB. In right ventricular hypertrophy, we can generally only estimate the influence on $\mathring{A}QRS_F$. In RBBB, the activation of the left and right ventricle occurs practically one after the other. Therefore, we do not consider the whole QRS but only the first 60–70 ms, so we get an approximate calculation of the $\mathring{A}QRS_F$. This is not always easy.

In LBBB, any calculation of the $\mathring{A}QRS_F$ is misleading and useless. An LBBB deforms the entire ventricular excitation so excessively that the amount of $\mathring{A}QRS_F$ that would be present without LBBB cannot be determined. We have made bad calculations ourselves, in contrast to a calculated $\mathring{A}QRS_F$ without LBBB.

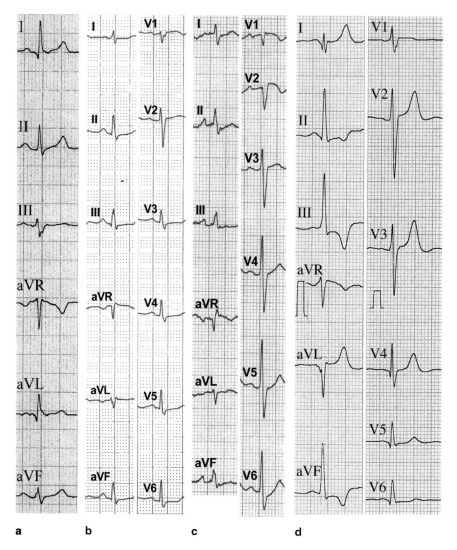

Figure 1.6 a. Frontal QRS axis (ÅQRS$_F$) = 0°. **b.** ÅQRS$_F$ = +80°. **c.** ÅQRS$_F$ = +120°.
d. ÅQRS$_F$ = +110°

In conclusion, the reader will soon recognize that ÅQRS$_F$ in the Einthoven leads
(I, II, III) does not fully coincide with ÅQRS$_F$ in the Goldberger leads (aVR, aVL,
aVF) and may differ between 5° and 15°. This means that ÅQRS$_F$ is always an
approximate value. Moreover, Einthoven's triangle is in fact not an isosceles triangle
but one with a shorter branch above, and with two longer branches, directed slightly
to the left, according to the mean frontal heart position (Figure 1.7).

Figure 1.7 Original and modified
Einthoven's triangle

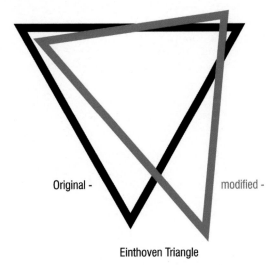

Original -   modified -

Einthoven Triangle

Chapter 2
Practical Approach

There are beginners in electrocardiogram (ECG) analysis who are fascinated by a special pattern (e.g., a bundle-branch block or a striking Q wave) and thereby overlook other abnormalities. The best way to avoid similar errors is to analyze an ECG systematically, step by step. However, for experienced ECG interpreters, loss of concentration can also occur for a variety of reasons (see Short Story).

Short Story

About 10 years ago, an ECG with obvious preexcitation (ECG 2.1), diagnosable by any dentist, was shown to the author by a very good-looking young colleague. The author's concentration was focused on the "wrong" subject and he interpreted the ECG as being normal.

Practical Approach

The practical approach includes:

- Analysis of rhythm
- Morphologic analysis of p, QRS, ST, and T (U) waves. The measurements of the PQ interval and of the QT (QTc) interval are included
- Definitive ECG diagnosis

ECG 2.1 Preexcitation with short PQ interval (0.10 s).
Obvious positive delta waves in III and aVF. Striking Q waves
(negative delta waves) in I and aVL and abnormal R waves in
V_1 and V_2

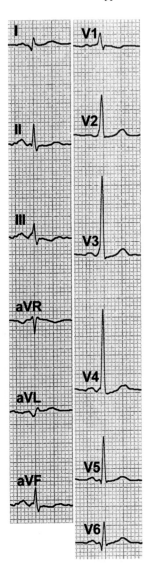

1. Analysis of rhythm

Step 1:   Rhythm regular or irregular?
   a. Regular: in most cases, normal SR
      Pathologic regular rhythms: *escape rhythms; some forms of supraventricular tachycardias; VT*
   b. Irregular: the most frequent cause of irregularity is regular SR *with supraventricular and ventricular premature beats. Complete irregularity of the R-R intervals: atrial fibrillation*

Step 2:   Normal (sinusal p) wave present? → SR. If not:
   a. Abnormal (nonsinusal) p waves present: *atrial rhythm*
   b. No p waves: *AV junctional rhythm*
   c. Replacement of p waves by *other atrial waves: atrial flutter or atrial fibrillation*

1. Analysis of rhythm (continued)

Step 3: Rate (of the ventricles)? Eventually rate of the abnormal (nonsinusal) p waves or flutter waves?

Step 4: PQ interval? If we measure the PQ interval, we will not only recognize a prolongation or shortening of the PQ time, but also the following:
   a. every p is conducted, or *not every p wave is conducted: in the 3 forms of AV block 2°*
   b. no p wave is conducted. *This means that atria and ventricles are working independently from each other, in the presence of AV block 3° = complete AV block*
   c. p waves are twisting around the QRS complexes: *in the special forms of AV dissociation*

Step 5: QRS duration normal (≤90 ms) or *prolonged*?
   QRS ≥120 ms: *pattern of BBB*
   a. Supraventricular rhythm/tachycardia *with aberration.*
   b. *Ventricular origin of the rhythm (with AV dissociation):*
      • *Low rate: ventricular escape rhythm*
      • *Medium rate: accelerated idioventricular rhythm*
      • *High rate: VT*

Note: Typical pathologic findings are italicized.
AV, atrioventricular; BBB, bundle-branch block; SR, sinus rhythm; VT, ventricular tachycardia.

2. Detailed analysis of morphology

Step 1: P
   1. Normal (sinusal)? (p duration 90–110 ms)
      Note: A negative p in lead I and (often) a positive p in lead aVR means "false poling" of the upper limb leads in 99% of the cases
   2. Pathologic p waves
   2a. p duration ≥110 ms, accentuated terminal negativity in lead V_1:
      Left atrial enlargement
   2b. p voltage ≥2.5 mm in leads III and aVF:*Right atrial enlargement*
   2c. Summation of 2a and 2b:*Biatrial enlargement*

Step 2: QRS
   1. Frontal QRS axis = ÅQRS$_F$? (DD of different ÅQRS$_F$ values, see Chapter 3)
   2. *Broad QRS?*
   2a. *Typical configuration for aberration: RBBB (QRS ≥120 ms) or LBBB (≥140 ms). More or less typical BBB (≥160 ms): suspicious for severe hyperkalemia.*
   2b. *Typical pattern of bilateral BBB (RBBB + LAFB or RBBB + LPFB)*
   2c. *Atypical BBB-like configuration (QRS ≥140 ms): suspicious for ventricular origin of rhythm, generally with AV dissociation*
   3. (Formally) pathologic Q or QS waves?
   3a. Typical for *old MI? (combined with symmetric negative T waves; typical history; risk factors for CHD)*
   3b. Atypical for old MI? (combined with asymmetric discordant T waves; atypical history; no risk factors for CHD)

DD:
   • Artifact: Q/QS in lead I; R/qR in lead aVR—false poling of limb leads (DD: *situs inversus*)
      • Normal variant: QS in lead III (Q$_{III}$)—attributable to projection
      • *LVH*
      • *Preexcitation (QS in III, aVF)*
      • *Hypertrophic (obstructive) cardiomyopathy*
      • *LBBB (QS in III, aVF, V_1 to V_4, with duration ≥140 ms)*

(continued)

2. Detailed analysis of morphology (continued)

    4. Signs of *LVH or RVH?* (Chapters 5 and 6)

    5. Signs of *LAFB or LPFB?* (Chapter 9)

    6. *Presence of delta wave?* (with shortened PQ: preexcitation)

    7. Presence of notching/slurring? DD: intraventricular conduction disturbance versus *normal variant*

    7a. Normal variant (Chapter 3)

    7b. *Pathologic, e.g., in old MI or left fascicular block* (Chapters 13 and 9, respectively)

Step 3:   ST

    1. ST elevation?

    1a. Normal variants: ST (in V_2/V_3), early repolarization (Chapter 3)

    1b. Pathologic:

      • Typical for *acute MI: consider other findings*; symptoms, history, risk factors for CHD (Chapter 13).

      • Typical for *acute pericarditis: frontal ST vector about +70°—ST elevations in leads aVF, II, and I* (Chapter 15).

      • Typical for *mirror image of ST depression: e.g., in LVH/systolic LV overload.*

    2. ST depression?

    2a. *Ischemic*

    2b. *LVH/LV overload*

    2c. *Related to BBB or other conditions* (Chapter 17)

Step 4:   T (and U)

    1. Asymmetric T negativity?

    1a. Normal in lead V_1; normal in vertical $\mathring{A}QRS_F$: in aVF, III(II); normal in left $\mathring{A}QRS_F$: in aVL.

    1b. Pathologic in *LVH/LV overload; preexcitation; BBB*

    2. Symmetric T negativity?

    2a. *Often ischemic*, but extensive DD

    2b. *Later stage of pericarditis; LVH/LV overload; acute pancreatitis; drugs; others*

    3. High and symmetric T?

    3a. *Ischemia* (rare, because short-lasting)

    3b. *Hyperkalemia*

    4. U negativity?

    4b. *Ischemic*; other conditions

Step 5:   QT

    1. QT prolonged

    1a. *Long QT syndromes*

    1b. *Hypocalcemia*

    2. QT shortened: *hypercalcemia*

    3. Fusion of T and U: *hypokalemia, long QT syndromes*

Step 6:   Definitive diagnosis

Note: Typical pathologic findings are italicized.

DD, differential diagnosis; $\mathring{A}QRS_F$, frontal QRS axis; AV, atrioventricular; BBB, bundle-branch block; CHD, coronary heart disease; LAFB, left anterior fascicular block; LPFB, left posterior fascicular block; LBBB, left bundle-branch block; RBBB, right bundle-branch block; LV, left ventricle; LVH, left ventricular hypertrophy; MI, myocardial infarction.

Definitive Electrocardiogram Diagnosis

Take the important normal and pathologic findings from the analysis above and put them into the following scheme:
Note: As mentioned above, an ECG must be interpreted in context with the clinical findings of a patient. Therefore, in this book, age and gender and the clinical diagnosis of the patient are provided for many ECG examples in the text.

	Example 1	*Example 2*
Rhythm/rate	SR, 72 beats/min	*Atrial fibrillation*, medium rate 90 beats/min (maximum 140 beats/min, minimum 40 beats/min)
p	Normal	–
PQ	Normal (0.16 s)	–
ÅQRS$_F$	(+80°)	LAD (−60°): *LAFB*
QRS	Normal	0.12 s, *LVH*
ST	Normal (elevation in V$_2$/V$_3$)	*Minor changes attributable to LAFB*
T	Normal(negative in III)	*Idem*
QT	Normal	Prolonged?
Special remarks	–	*Fusion of T and U*
Diagnosis	Normal ECG	*Atrial fibrillation, LAFB, LVH,* Hypokalemia?

Note: Typical pathologic findings are italicized.
LAD, left axis deviation; LAFB, left anterior fascicular block; LVH, left ventricular hypertrophy; SR, sinus rhythm.

Chapter 3
The Normal Electrocardiogram and Its (Normal) Variants

Knowledge about the normal electrocardiogram (ECG) and its (normal) variants is enormously important because, when a physician looks at a new ECG, he or she automatically compares it with the normal ECGs stored *visually* in the posterior part and *intellectually* in the frontal part of the cerebrum. Therefore, in this chapter, normal components of the ECG and its variants are discussed so that the reader can make accurate comparisons.

Components of the Normal Electrocardiogram

Sinus Rhythm

The sinus node produces the normal rhythm of the whole heart, resulting in a p wave with the typical atrial vectors (Figure 3.1a and b). Because the sinus node is localized in the right atrium (high laterally at the entry of the superior vena cava), the right atrium is activated first and the left atrium approximately 20 ms later, resulting in a fusion of two p waves, both forming the normal p wave. Its duration is 0.09–0.11 s, best measured in lead II where the beginning and the end of the p wave are clearly visible in most cases.

In the frontal plane, the p wave is positive on all leads except in aVL (where it is negative or biphasic +/−) and in, III, where it may be biphasic +/−. In the horizontal plane, the p wave is only biphasic in V_1 (because the left atrial vector is directed posteriorly and to the left), with a longer part of the (first) positive component than the (second) negative part. In all other precordial leads (V_2 to V_6), the normal p wave is positive. The normal rate of sinus rhythm is 60–100 beats/min (or perhaps better, 50–90 beats/min) (see ECG 3.1). Rates higher than 90–100 beats/min are called sinus tachycardia (normal in emotion and on exercise) and rates less than 50–60 beats/min are called sinus bradycardia (normal in many individuals at rest, especially athletes).

Alterations of the normal p wave are discussed in Chapter 4, "Atrial Enlargement and Other Abnormalities of the p Wave" and in the chapters about arrhythmias.

M. Gertsch, *The ECG Manual: An Evidence-Based Approach*,
© Springer-Verlag London Limited 2009

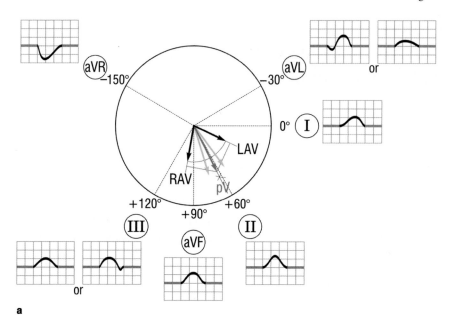

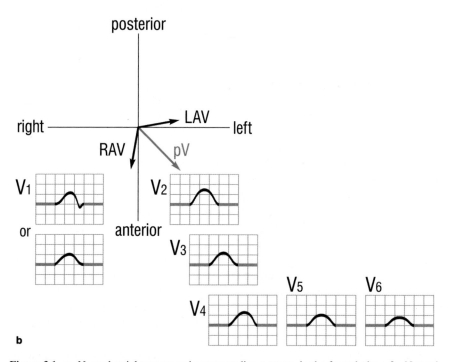

Figure 3.1 a. Normal atrial vectors and corresponding p waves in the frontal plane. **b.** Normal atrial vectors and corresponding p waves in the horizontal plane. RAV, right atrial vector; LAV, left atrial vector; pV, p vector

ECG 3.1 Normal sinus rhythm (81 beats/min)

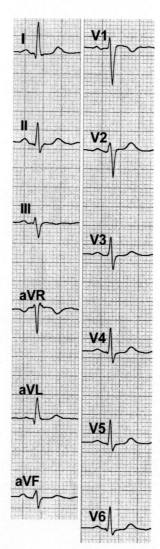

PQ Interval

The normal PQ interval measures 0.13–0.20 s (in sinus bradycardia up to 0.21 s) and is determined from the beginning of the p wave to the beginning of the QRS complex.

Prolonged PQ intervals (≥0.21 s) were found in 8% of males and 12% of females. In young, healthy students, a 2° atrioventricular block of the Wenckebach type (see Chapter 12, "Atrioventricular Block and Atrioventricular Dissociation") was detected in 6% of males and 4% of females.

QRS Complex

The QRS complex is quite variable in the frontal plane and largely dependent on the individual's age. Table 3.1 shows the common frontal QRS axis ($\mathring{A}QRS_F$) for approximately 70% of normal individuals. ECG 3.2a–g shows the typical $\mathring{A}QRS_F$ for a variety of ages. A sudden change of $\mathring{A}QRS_F$ to the left is rare (perhaps occurring in inferior infarction or in a new left anterior fascicular block), but a sudden change of $\mathring{A}QRS_F$ to the right can be seen in acute pulmonary embolism.

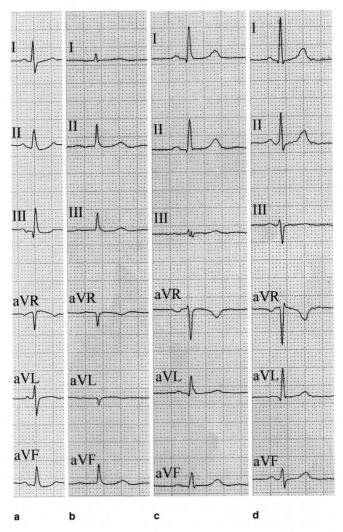

ECG 3.2 a–d Different frontal QRS axis ($\mathring{A}QRS_F$) values by age. **a.** 18-year-old, $\mathring{A}QRS_F$ +80°. **b.** 25-year-old, $\mathring{A}QRS_F$ +75°. **c.** 40-year-old, $\mathring{A}QRS_F$ +30°. **d.** 54-year-old, $\mathring{A}QRS_F$ +20°

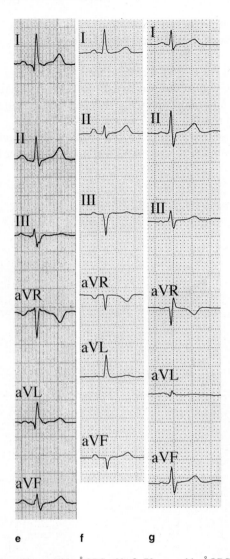

e   f   g

ECG 3.2 (continued) **e.** 60-year-old, ÅQRS$_F$ 0°. **f.** 73-year-old, ÅQRS$_F$ –20°. **g.** 25-year-old, ÅQRS$_F$ not determinable. The positive and negative components of the QRS complex have almost the same amplitude in the individual limb leads. This frontal QRS axis is called *sagittal axis*

In contrast to the frontal plane in the horizontal plane, the QRS complex generally is characterized by a striking uniformity. In leads V$_1$ and V$_2$, we find an rS complex, a small r and a deep S, especially in V$_2$. In lead V$_3$, the transition zone begins—a change from a predominantly negative to a predominantly positive QRS complex. Therefore, in lead V$_3$, the R wave can have almost the same amplitude as the S wave. From V$_4$ to V$_6$, the QRS is positive, with an Rs complex; leads V$_5$ and V$_6$ often have a small initial deflection, forming a qRs complex.

Clockwise and Counterclockwise Rotation
in the Horizontal Plane (in the Precordial Leads)

A clockwise rotation (ECG 3.3), a shift of the QRS transition zone to the left, is rarer in a normal ECG than the contrary. In pathologic situations, it is seen, for example, in anterior myocardial infarction, left anterior fascicular block, and (often forgotten) in marked right and/or left ventricular dilatation.

A counterclockwise rotation (ECG 3.4) is frequent in younger persons and especially in children. Even the R wave in V_2 might have a greater amplitude than the

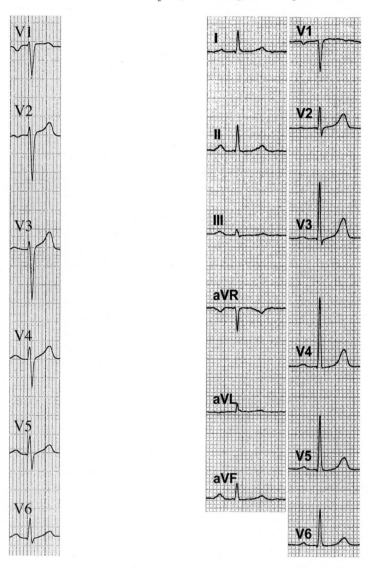

ECG 3.3 Clockwise rotation of QRS   **ECG 3.4** Counterclockwise rotation

S wave in children (in 10%), whereas this is rare in adults (only 1%). A tall R wave in V_1 is frequent in young children and is found in 20% at ages 8–10 and in 10% at ages 12–16, without right ventricular hypertrophy. In adults, a great (and relative broad) R wave in V_1 is encountered, for example, in one type of preexcitation, in posterior myocardial infarction, and occasionally in severe mitral stenosis.

Puzzling Normal Variants Caused by Projection

Q_{III}

Occasionally, we find a QR (ECG 3.5), Qr, or even a QS complex in lead III, but much rarer in aVF. In the absence of a previous inferior infarction, the T waves are generally positive and asymmetric.

QS in V_2/V_3

Rarely, a QS complex in V_2 and or V_3 could imitate an anteroseptal infarction (ECG 3.6), even with correctly attached leads. Anamnestic and clinical findings and an echo will resolve the problem.

Pseudo-Preexcitation

An exquisite projection of the first 20-ms ventricular vector, generally in the inferior leads III and aVF and in the precordial transition zone, leads to a pseudo-delta wave (ECG 3.7a and b). However, the normal variant can be recognized by the normal PQ interval.

S_I/S_{II}/S_{III} Type

This frontal QRS type is occasionally seen in the so-called sagittal type, rarely in right ventricular hypertrophy, and has no significance (ECG 3.8).

Pseudo-Notching or Pseudo-Slurring

The projection of normal ventricular vectors on certain leads may lead to notching or slurring (Figure 3.2a and b) that could be confounded with an intraventricular conduction disturbance. However, pseudo-notching (not different from slurring) is only encountered in the inferior frontal leads III and aVF or in the precordial transition zone (ECG 3.9), which means it is restricted to one, or maximally two, precordial leads.

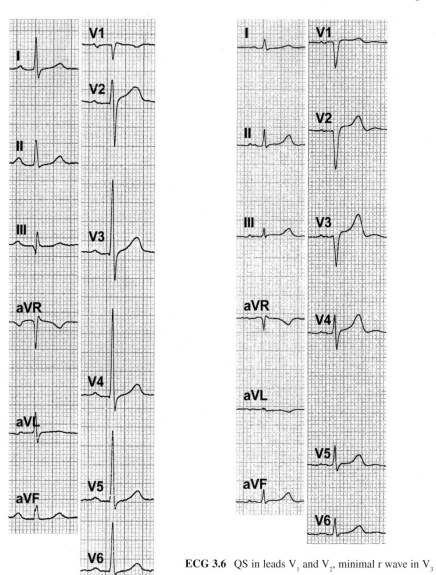

ECG 3.6 QS in leads V_1 and V_2, minimal r wave in V_3

ECG 3.5 Q_{III}

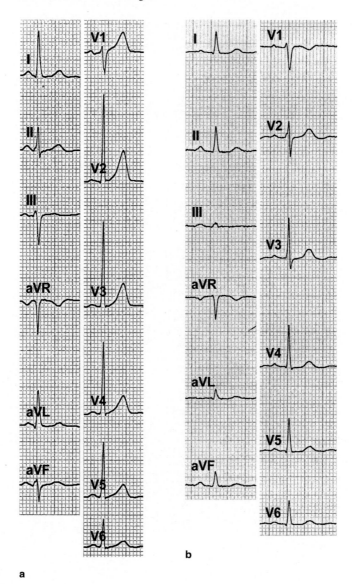

ECG 3.7 a. Pseudo-delta wave in lead II. **b.** Pseudo-delta wave in lead V$_2$

ECG 3.8 $S_I/S_{II}/S_{III}$ type

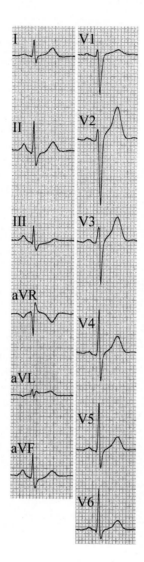

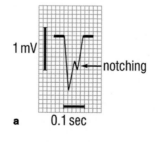

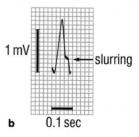

Figure 3.2 a. Notching of QRS. **b.** Slurring of QRS

ECG 3.9 Pseudo-notching in transition zone, leads V$_3$ and III

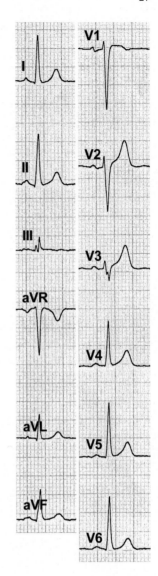

Other Normal Variants

False Poling of the Upper Limbs

Erroneous exchange of the arm leads is by far the most frequent. We encounter an inverted QRS complex in lead I with a striking Q wave, also with inversion of the T wave, and, of coarse, always a negative p wave (ECG 3.10). The consequences

ECG 3.10 False poling of the upper limb leads

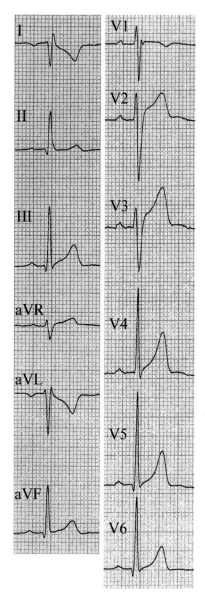

for the other limb leads are manifold (changing by different frontal QRS axes). However, a glance at the precordial leads excludes a myocardial infarction, and corrected placement of the limb leads results in an accurate ECG.

Incomplete Right Bundle-Branch Block

Incomplete right bundle-branch block is found mainly in young people with a healthy heart (ECG 3.11). It is a mandatory sign in ASD II (atrial septal defect of the ostium secundum type), where r′ is generally higher (and broader) than the first r wave. It may also be present in a healthy individual. More significant for ASD II is a negative T in V_2 (but rarely up to V_4/V_5).

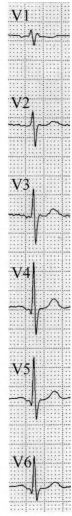

ECG 3.11 Incomplete right bundle-branch block with r > r′ in V_1. It is better to consider the product of amplitude × duration of the r and r′ than the amplitude alone

ST Segment

Osborn Wave

We delegate the Osborn wave to the variations of the ST segment. It is a very short, positive deflection, measuring ≤1 mm and arising just at the end of QRS and the beginning of ST, in the limb leads and especially in leads V_4 to V_6. The Osborn wave is always present in hypothermic hearts (at open-heart surgery in hypothermia, ECG 3.12a), in approximately 30%–40% of acute pericarditis cases (where it is called "stork-leg sign"), and occasionally in early repolarization. As a normal variant, it is found rarely in its "mini-form" in leads V_3 to V_6 as a completely harmless variation (ECG 3.12b).

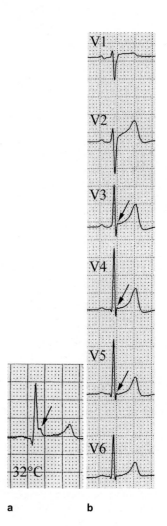

ECG 3.12 a. Temperature 32°C. **b.** Small Osborn wave, without ST elevation, in leads V_4 to V_6 (arrow)

a   b

ST Elevation in V_2

For many physicians, an ST elevation above 1 mm is equal to myocardial ischemia, especially in combination with thoracic pain. However, the ST segment is always elevated 1 mm or more in lead V_2 (up to 2–3 mm, especially in sinus bradycardia), and less in V_3. The Short Story demonstrates the possible consequences of a misinterpretation of this fact.

Short Story/Case Report

A 38-year-old man with acute pain at the left side of the thorax is seen at the emergency station. He mentions having a subfebrile body temperature in the past several days. His only risk factor for coronary heart disease is that one uncle had a myocardial infarction at the age of 50. His blood pressure is 150/90 mmHg. The ECG shows sinus bradycardia with ST elevation of 2–2.5 mm in leads V_2 and V_3 (ECG 3.13). Creatine kinase (CK) is slightly elevated (by 20%); myocardial fraction of CK and troponin are normal. There is leucocytosis of 11,000. The diagnosis of acute anterior infarction is made and a thrombolysis is performed. The ECG remains unchanged. The pain disappears after the first dose of morphine and blood pressure normalizes. One day later, the diagnosis is revised and an infectious disease of uncertain origin with pain of the chest skeletal muscle is presumed. The patient insists on a coronary angiography. The coronary arteries are normal. The next day, the patient is without symptoms and is discharged with aspirin 500 mg for 7 days. On the basis of serum reactions positive for coxsackie virus, the final diagnosis of coxsackie infection with muscle pain is made.

Conclusion: The chest pain was atypical and the ECG normal. The slightly elevated CK was overestimated. It would have been better to observe the patient for several hours and to control the ECG and the enzymes.

Early Repolarization

This variation is not well defined. Generally, it means a significant ST elevation of several millimeters arising from the R wave on the inferior or anterolateral leads (ECG 3.14), formally completely imitating acute myocardial infarction (or Prinzmetal angina). However, the finding is *constant*, which means it does not show any evolution to infarction, the patient is generally young, and has neither angina nor risk factors for coronary heart disease.

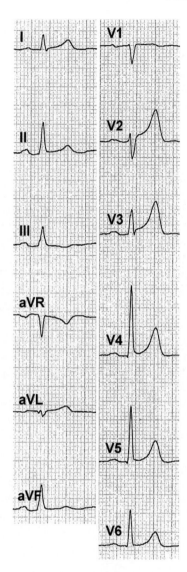

ECG 3.13 ST elevation of V_2/V_3 (V_4) in 38-year-old man described in the Short Story

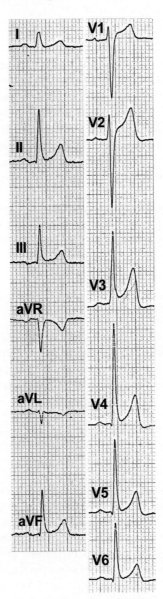

ECG 3.14 Early repolarization. ST elevation of 2 mm, arising from the R waves in V_3 to V_4 (V_5/V_6)

T Wave and U Wave

The T wave represents the most frequently variable part of the ECG, in normal and pathologic conditions (for the latter, see Chapter 17, "Alterations of Repolarization"). In the normal ECG, the T wave is positive in all limb leads except in aVR and may be biphasic +/− in III/aVF and aVL (never in I!), or even negative in III/aVF.

In the precordial leads, the T wave is positive in all leads except V_1, where it is often biphasic +/−. In V_2, a negative T wave is always pathologic, indicating a disease of the right heart or a mirror image of acute strictly posterior myocardial infarction. Rarely, young individuals up to 30 years may show a negative T in V_2 of no significance.

The U waves (that are thought to represent the repolarization of the Purkinje fibers) may be normally positive, flat, or absent. Negative U waves have been described in ischemia or in severe aortic valve incompetence.

QT Duration

A QT prolongation of more than 10% of the normal QT [or better, QT_C = rate-corrected QT duration, corresponding to the Bazett formula: $QTc = QT/\sqrt{60}/rate = QT\ (ms)/\sqrt{R\text{-}R}\ (ms)$] is pathologic (see chapter Alterations of Repolarization). A shortened QT duration is rare, often indicating hypercalcemia.

Arrhythmias

It is difficult if not impossible to classify many arrhythmias into normal variants and pathologic findings. We know, for example, that episodes of ventricular tachycardia or a slow ventricular escape rhythm may be found in apparently healthy individuals, especially athletes. However, no physician would classify a ventricular tachycardia or a ventricular rate of 35 beats/min as a normal variant. Both examples represent clinically important and often dangerous arrhythmias that may arise rarely in healthy individuals under special conditions and in these cases are likely harmless.

However, in individuals without heart disease, there is a substantial number of arrhythmias that may represent normal variants. In most cases, the three following conditions must be fulfilled:

1. Absence of any heart disease
2. Exclusion of many arrhythmias *not* representing normal variants, meaning pathologic findings (Table 3.2)
3. A normal variant arrhythmia should occur only rarely and not be associated with a very low or high ventricular rate.

Table 3.1 Frequent normal variant arrhythmias

- Sinus bradycardia (minimal rate approximately
  45 beats/min; minimal instantaneous rate during sleep approximately 35 beats/min)
- Sinus tachycardia (maximal rate approximately 110 beats/min)
- Sinus arrhythmia
- Isolated ventricular pauses <2 s during sleep
- Isolated AV-junctional (AV-nodal) escape beats (during sinus arrhythmia or after a PB)
- Short episodes of AV-nodal rhythm (with retrograde atrial activation)
- Short episodes (<10 beats?) of "AV dissociation" (with accrochage, with synchronization)
- Short episodes of accelerated idionodal rhythm
- Episodes of normocardic ectopic atrial rhythm (e.g., so-called coronary sinus rhythm)
- Supraventricular PBs (in most cases atrial PBs), if:
  a. Isolated (<200/24 h?)
  b. Less than 5 salvos (or <20?) of maximal 3 beats
  c. Instantaneous rate (beat-to-beat interval) <160 beats/min
  d. Isolated early atrial PBs with functional complete AV block
- VPBs, if:
  a. Isolated (<200/24 hours?)
  b. Monomorphic
  c. Isolated "couplets" (<20/24 hours?), instantaneous rate <160 beats/min
  d. Isolated VPBs with "pseudo-R on T phenomenon" (VPB after 90% of the preceding
     QT interval: "supernormal period").

AV, atrioventricular; PB, premature beat; VPB, ventricular premature beat.

Table 3.2 Arrhythmias not representing normal variants = pathologic findings

- Complete AV block
- AV block 2°, type Mobitz and type "high degree"
- Sinoatrial block 2° and 3°
- Ventricular pauses of >2-s duration
- Monomorphic VT (>3 ventricular beats)
- Polymorphic VT (torsades de pointes, other forms)
- Ventricular triplets (3 consecutive VPBs), multiple couplets
- Multiple ventricular couplets
- Single VPBs, if:
  a. >200/24 hours?
  b. Polymorphic
  c. With true R on T phenomenon (VPB before 90% of the preceding
  T wave: potential vulnerable period)
- Most forms of supraventricular tachycardias
  (such as atrial flutter, atrial fibrillation, reentrant
  AV tachycardias, reentry tachycardias in the
  Wolff-Parkinson-White syndrome)
- Supraventricular PBs in salvos (>3 beats) and at a
  high rate (>160/min).
- Rare arrhythmias such as parasystole, accelerated
  idioventricular rhythm, and AV dissociation with interference
- Lastly, of course, ventricular fibrillation

AV, atrioventricular; VT, ventricular tachycardia; PB, premature beat; VPB, ventricular premature beat.

Table 3.1 lists the arrhythmias that often represent normal variants. The number of normal supraventricular premature beats (PBs) and especially of normal ventricular PBs is as arbitrary as questionable. Normal variant arrhythmias may be *felt* by an individual person. Table 3.2 shows arrhythmias that never represent normal variants.

Day-to-Day Variations and Circadian Variations

These variations may be interesting but have little clinical importance and may be neglected.

Conclusion

As mentioned at the beginning of this chapter, every "unusual" ECG pattern should be interpreted in context with the conditions of the investigated person, including age, anamnestic and other clinical findings, and quality of symptoms.

Chapter 4
Atrial Enlargement and Other Abnormalities of the p Wave

Pathologic p waves in sinus rhythm (SR) are not as serious as QRS alterations. However, abnormal p waves may give some insight into hemodynamic abnormalities, especially if they are associated with pathologic QRS complexes.

The classical p mitrale, p pulmonale, and p biatriale are attributable to chronic overload of the left, right, or both atria, with consecutive hypertrophy and dilatation (enlargement) of the respective atria. In general, left atrial enlargement is used as a synonym for p mitrale, right atrial enlargement for p pulmonale, and biatrial enlargement for p biatriale.

Left Atrial Enlargement (p Mitrale)

The longer-lasting activation of the hypertrophic left atrium (LA) provokes prolongation (≥0.110 ms) and sometimes bifidity of the p wave, especially in leads I or II and V_6, with an interpeak distance of >40 ms. The second and negative portion of the p wave in lead V_1 (and often V_2) is accentuated (ECGs 4.1 and 4.2).

Several decades ago, classical "p mitrale," often with clear bifidity, was frequently encountered in patients with mitral stenosis (ECG 4.1). In many countries, the (electrocardiogram) ECG pattern was used in attempt to **decrease** rheumatic fever. The pattern of LA enlargement, often with less clear bifidity, was more often found in severe mitral valve incompetence of any etiology, in aortic valve diseases, and in hypertensive and other heart diseases with chronic left atrial overload.

In newer publications, the ECG pattern of LA enlargement is compared with LA dimension, in mitral and aortic valve diseases. The specificity of the ECG pattern is high (approximately 90%), whereas the sensitivity is modest (30%–60%). A bifid p wave is a rare finding, and in patients with LA diameter ≥60 mm, atrial fibrillation is present in approximately 70%.

In the elderly, p prolongation may be attributable to intraatrial conduction disturbance and is not necessarily associated with LA enlargement. In general, major LA enlargement predisposes one to atrial fibrillation, thrombosis in the LA (especially in the appendage), and consecutive cerebral stroke.

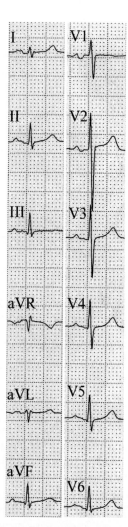

ECG 4.1 Electrocardiogram obtained from a 56-year-old woman with severe mitral stenosis. p Mitrale/left atrium (LA) enlargement: PQ duration 120 ms, bifidity of p waves in limb leads, V_6 (V_2 to V_5); accentuated and prolonged negative terminal portion of p in lead V_1. Echo: LA diameter 65 mm

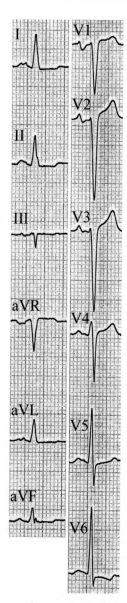

ECG 4.2 Electrocardiogram obtained from a 34-year-old man with hypertensive cardiomyopathy. p Mitrale/left atrium enlargement: PQ duration 120 ms, p bifidity in aVL, V_3 to V_5. Accentuated terminal p negativity in V_1/V_2

Right Atrial Enlargement (p Pulmonale)

Because activation of the right atrium (RA) begins earlier than that of the LA, an increase of the right atrial vector does not prolong the p duration. p Pulmonale is characterized by tall and sometimes pointed p waves in leads II, aVF, and III (ECG 4.3). The amplitude of the p waves is >2.5 mm in at least one of these leads. In the opposite lead aVL, the p wave is completely negative. The p wave may be higher than normal and pointed in leads V_1 and V_2.

The classical p pulmonale (as defined above) is rare and is found in patients with lung diseases, especially chronic obstructive pulmonary disease. A p wave amplitude of 2.0–2.5 mm in lead II is frequent and can represent RA enlargement of minor

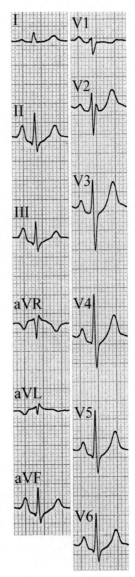

ECG 4.3 Electrocardiogram obtained from a 54-year-old man with chronic obstructive pulmonary disease. p Pulmonale/right atrium enlargement: prominent and peaked p waves in II (3 mm), aVF, and III. Peaked p waves also in V_2/V_3 and atypically prominent in V_4 to V_6. Note the unusual "PQ depression," as in early acute pericarditis, caused by the enhanced opposite atrial repolarization vector (Ta)

degree, or, more often, a normal variant especially in young asthenic individuals, and in elevated sympathic tone (with sinus tachycardia).

Biatrial Enlargement (p Biatriale)

Biatrial enlargement is very rare and combines the criteria of left and right atrial hypertrophy/dilatation (ECG 4.4). p Biatriale can be seen in combined severe diseases of heart and lung, and in patients with complex congenital heart disease.

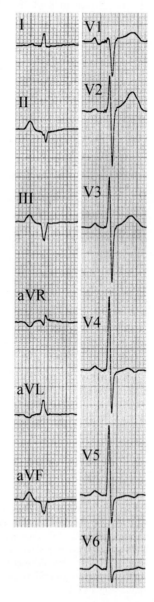

ECG 4.4 Electrocardiogram obtained from a 58-year-old man with coronary heart disease with old inferior and posterior myocardial infarction, chronic obstructive pulmonary disease. p Biatriale/biatrial enlargement: 1. Peaky and high p waves in inferior leads, p ≥2.5 mm in II. 2. p Duration 120 ms, accentuated terminal p negativity in V_1. The QS (or rSr'?) configuration in the inferior leads and the broad/tall R waves in V_2 are the result of infarction

Acute Left Atrial Overload

Although the borderline between left atrial overload without and with hypertrophy
is not clearly established, it is reasonable to define the p pattern of left atrial overload without hypertrophy. Acute left atrial overload (or chronic overload without
hypertrophy) is characterized by a normal p duration, combined with accentuated
p negativity in lead V_1 (the negative component of the p wave being greater than
the positive one). This pattern is common in many diseases leading to left atrial
overload such as hypertension and aortic and mitral valve diseases of moderate
degree. It is often present during the acute stage of myocardial infarction (ECG 4.5)
and generally regresses during the following days. The pattern may also be attributable to incorrect placement of lead V_1 (and V_2), one intercostal space too high.

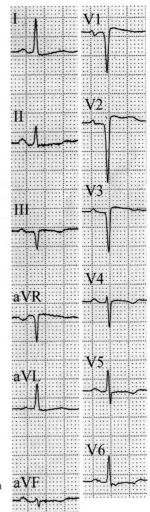

ECG 4.5 Electrocardiogram obtained from a 70-year-old
woman. Two-day-old anteroseptal myocardial infarction (MI).
Acute left atrial overload: p duration 100–110 ms. Slightly
accentuated terminal p negativity in lead V_1, with normalization
after 2 days (QS complexes and ST elevation in V_1 to V_3 as a
result of MI)

Acute Right Atrial Overload

Acute right atrial overload (e.g., in acute pulmonary embolism) leads to only minor (or no) alterations of the p wave in most cases. A peaked p wave in lead V_1 or V_2 might be the only evidence for it. A classical p pulmonale in this condition is very rare.

Other Abnormalities of the p Wave

Negative p Wave in Lead I

A negative p wave in lead I is caused by false poling of limb leads (exchange of the arm leads; see Chapter 3) in 99%, and in 1% by left atrial rhythm. False poling also leads to a Q wave in lead I. However, a glance at the precordial leads will clarify that there is no anterior infarction. For all possibilities of false poling, see M. Gertsch, *The ECG*, Springer, 2004.

Right Atrial Enlargement in Chronic Pulmonary Hypertension of Purely Vascular Origin

In vascular pulmonary hypertension caused by chronic pulmonary embolism, intake of aminorectic drugs, or in the form of unknown etiology, we miss the classical pattern of "p pulmonale" (p pulmonale parenchymal). However, we find a p wave with the greatest amplitude in lead II and an amplitude equal or greater in lead I than in lead III. Additionally, there are prominent p waves in some of the precordial leads ("p pulmonale vasculare"; ECG 4.6).

ECG 4.6 Electrocardiogram obtained from a 48-year-old woman with so-called "p pulmonale vasculare": primary pulmonary hypertension. Giant p wave in lead II. Note that the p wave in lead I is higher than in lead III and that the p wave in aVL is flat positive. Peaked p waves in lead V_1 up to V_6. Surprisingly, frontal QRS axis is +20° and signs of right ventricular hypertrophy are lacking

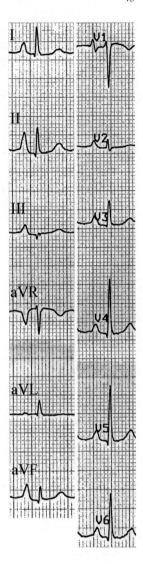

Atrial Infarction

In very rare cases, atrial infarction may induce a deformation of the p wave together with a positive or negative segment between the end of the p wave and the beginning of QRS.

Rare Conditions of Atrial Enlargement

In tricuspid atresia, a condition with extreme right atrial overload, the p wave may be negative in lead V_1. In Ebstein's anomaly, giant p waves in the inferior leads, combined with alterations of the QRS complex and repolarization, may be encountered. Hyperkalemia rarely produces a classical p pulmonale. Interesting for vectorial reasons, left atrial overload can imitate p pulmonale, if the left atrial vector is abnormally projected to the inferior leads, with the second part of the p wave being higher than the first one. A glance to lead V_1 allows the diagnosis of left atrial overload and clinical findings confirm the correct interpretation.

Abnormal p Waves in Arrhythmias

Abnormal p waves as a result of rhythm disturbances are of great interest. The conditions are discussed in Chapters 18–20, 23, and 24.

Chapter 5
Left Ventricular Hypertrophy

Left ventricular hypertrophy (LVH) is a common pathologic finding. Approximately 20% of the population of 50-year-olds, with an increasing percentage in older people, experience LVH. It represents an independent predictor of premature death, which is about as clinically important as frequent ventricular premature beats. The enhanced risk is attributed to consecutive malignant ventricular arrhythmias and to heart failure. It is possible to prevent or reduce LVH with drugs such as angiotensin-converting enzyme inhibitors, thus eliminating or diminishing the fatal consequences. Therefore, the reliable diagnosis of LVH has gained increased interest during the last two decades.

Etiology and Prevalence

The most common etiology of LVH is arterial hypertension. Other etiologies include aortic valve diseases, hypertrophic cardiomyopathies, and multiple rare diseases such as the metabolic disorders of hyperthyreosis, Cushing's disease, and acromegalia. LVH probably represents the most common pathologic condition with potentially severe consequences.

LVH is detected more frequently by echocardiography than by electrocardiography. There are several reasons for this fact:

- The echo classifies all patients in whom left ventricular mass exceeds the normal value ($134\,g/m^2$ for male, $119\,g/m^2$ for female, in our institution) as hypertrophic, including numerous cases with borderline and minor LVH. On the basis of this definition, in the Framingham study, the prevalence of LVH was 16% in men and 19% in women; at the age of 70 or older, up to 33% in men and 49% in women. In another population of 3338 persons with uncomplicated hypertension, LVH was found in 12% of people with mild hypertension and in 20% of patients with moderate hypertension.
- Electrocardiography, as a highly indirect method, generally detects only medium and severe LVH—the grades with the most important clinical consequences. However, the electrocardiogram (ECG) is influenced by habitus, body mass,

age, gender, and heart position. Also, the frontal QRS axis is variable, thus compromising the value of some ECG indices. None of these factors are an issue in echocardiography.

• In the diagnosis of LVH, the ECG excels, with an excellent specificity with most indices, but at the expense of a low sensitivity. In contrast, the echo can diagnose *and* exclude LVH with the same accuracy.

In comparative echo studies, generally only one ECG criterion was used, and often not the best one.

Pathophysiology and Its Influence on the Electrocardiogram

Generally, systolic overload of the left ventricle, for example, in hypertension, induces hypertrophy of the ventricle. Thereafter, left ventricular dilatation develops, together with dilatation and hypertrophy of the left atrium.

In diastolic overload, which is rare, dilatation occurs first and hypertrophy later. In systolic overload, astonishingly, the first sign in the ECG is often an accentuated negativity of the second part of the p wave in lead V_1, indicating left atrial overload. Thereafter, the left ventricular muscle thickens, in order to overcome the increased vascular resistance. Without therapy, dilatation follows, with the danger of consecutive heart failure and ventricular arrhythmias. With the ECG, generally only hypertrophy that manifests in an increase of the R wave voltage, often combined with negative asymmetric T waves, can be diagnosed. Dilatation is rarely diagnosable, but it can be suspected by a QRS clockwise rotation in the precordial leads.

"Pure" patterns of diastolic overload are extremely rare, found, for example, in patent ductus Botalli and in the early stage of aortic incompetence. In most other cases, the common pattern of LVH is found.

Today, echocardiography is generally acknowledged as a preferable diagnostic method with a specificity *and* sensitivity of approximately 90%, compared with anatomic evaluation using the left ventricular dissecting method as the golden standard. However, the ECG can and should be used as a screening method. Why?

First, the specificity of the frequently used ECG criteria is equal to the echo, at 90%–95%, although at the expense of sensitivity, which is poor, at 20%–35%. However, it must be remembered that the high specificity is only valid for individuals older than 40 years. Second, generally, an ECG is still performed at least 10 times more often than an echocardiogram, and it is done for different purposes. Thus, the detection of LVH is possible at the same time. Third, the ECG can be registered by a technical assistant or a nurse within a short time and interpreted by the physician within several minutes. Finally, the costs of an ECG are only about 15% of the costs of an echo. How then to proceed in practice?

Electrocardiogram Indices for Left Ventricular Hypertrophy

If one or two of the older voltage ECG indices (summarized in Table 5.1) *and* the recently published Cornell index (Table 5.2) are positive in a patient older than 40 years, LVH can be diagnosed with great accuracy. However, if all these indices are negative, a diagnosis of LVH cannot be excluded. In patients with hypertension or other diseases disposing to LVH, an echocardiogram must be performed. In young patients, the ECG voltage criteria may be false positive. In doubtful cases, in consideration of the clinical conditions, an echo is useful.

Other, older ECG indices, not mentioned in Table 5.1, which also include T wave negativity or the behavior of the p wave in lead V_1, have not improved the detection or exclusion of LVH (for example, the relatively complex Romhilt point score index).

ECGs 5.1 and 5.2 show examples of LVH with predominantly positive voltage criteria, and ECG 5.3 shows LVH and negative voltage criteria. As mentioned previously, a false negative result is a frequent finding, indicating low sensitivity. ECG 5.4 is an example of a false-positive Sokolow index. This finding is quite rare at age 40 years or older. However, it is not so rare in healthy, young individuals, especially in men.

Table 5.1 Previous electrocardiogram voltage indices for detection of left ventricular hypertrophy

a. Limb leads
- $R_{aVL} \geq 11\,mm$ (>12 mm) (Sokolow/Lyon II)
- $R_{aVF} \geq 20\,mm$
- $R_I + S_{III} \geq 25\,mm$ (Gubner/Ungerleider)
- $R_I - R_{III} + S_{III} - S_I \geq 17\,mm$ (Lewis, 1914!)
- $R_{aVF} \geq 24\,mm$

b. Precordial leads
- $S_{V1} + R_{V5}$ (or R_{V6}) $\geq 35\,mm$ (Sokolow = Sokolow/Lyon I)
- R_{V5} (or V_6) $\geq 26\,mm$
- $S_{V2} + S_{V3} \geq 35\,mm$
- $S_{V1} \geq 24\,mm$
- $(R + S_{V3}) + (R + S_{V4}) \geq 32\,mm$
- $(R + S)_{maximal\ precordial} \geq 45\,mm$

Table 5.2 Cornell indices for detection of left ventricular hypertrophy

a. Cornell index
- $R_{aVL} + S_{V3} \geq 28\,mm$ (male)
- $R_{aVL} + S_{V3} \geq 20\,mm$ (female)

b. Cornell product (mm × s)
- Male: $(R_{aVL} + S_{V3}) \times$ QRS duration
- Female: $(R_{aVL} + S_{V3} + 8\,mm) \times$ QRS duration (female)

c. Corrected Cornell product
- Male: $(R_{aVL} + S_{V3}) + [0.0174 \times (age - 49)] + [0.191 \times (BMI - 26.5)]$
- Female: $(R_{aVL} + S_{V3}) + [0.0387 \times (age - 50)] + [0.212 \times (BMI - 24.9)]$

BMI, body mass index.

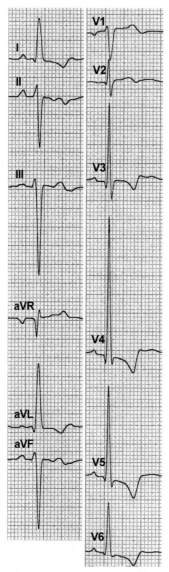

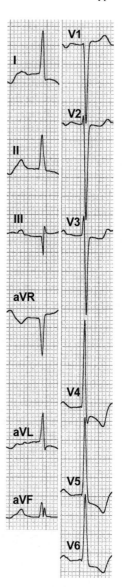

ECG 5.1 Electrocardiogram obtained from a 53-year-old man with severe left ventricular hypertrophy (LVH), 1 year after aortic valve replacement for aortic valve incompetence. Positive voltage indices: 1. $R_{aVL} = 15\,mm$ (>11 mm); 2. $R_I + S_{III} = 31\,mm$ (>25 mm). Negative voltage indices: 1. Cornell, 21 mm (>28 mm for male); 2. Sokolow ($S_I + R_{V5}$) = 29 mm (>35 mm). Plus: negative T waves in leads with tall R waves. Left axis deviation caused by LVH, probably not the result of left anterior fascicular block. Echo: left ventricular mass index 270 g/m^2

ECG 5.2 Electrocardiogram obtained from a 69-year-old woman with left ventricular hypertrophy, 2 months after aortic valve replacement. Positive voltage indices: Sokolow, 41 mm; Cornell, 30 mm (20 mm for female). Negative voltage indices: $R_{aVL} = 9\,mm$; $R_{V1} + S_{III}$ = 19 mm. Plus: significant ST depression and T inversion in anterolateral leads. Echo: left ventricular mass index 150 g/m^2

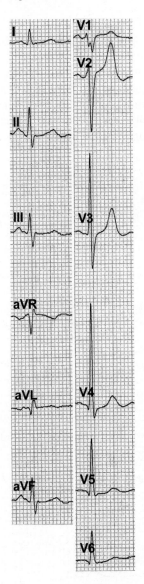

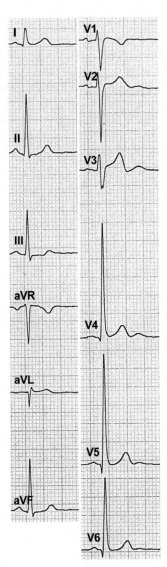

ECG 5.3 Electrocardiogram obtained from an 80-year-old man. All usual voltage criteria are negative. Left ventricular hypertrophy is suspected from the tall RS complexes in V_3/V_4, about 30 mm each. Hypertensive and coronary heart disease. Echo: left ventricular mass 165 g/m^2

ECG 5.4 Electrocardiogram obtained from a 24-year-old man. Positive Sokolow index (37 mm); all other voltage indices negative. Echo: no left ventricular hypertrophy. False-positive Sokolow index in a young, healthy individual

The Cornell index, a more recent voltage criterion, accounts for gender: $R_{aVL} + S_{V3} \geq 28$ mm in men and ≥ 20 mm in women (see Table 5.2, and ECGs 5.1–5.4). The specificity of this index is 80%–90%, and the sensitivity is approximately 35%. With the Cornell product, which is the product of the Cornell voltage, and the QRS duration (Table 5.2), the sensitivity could be improved from 35% to 51%.

In the very rare pattern of diastolic overload, the following signs are typical: thin but high R waves, a slightly elevated ST segment in the lateral leads (ST elevation in leads V_1 and V_2 is a normal finding), and high, almost symmetric, positive T waves (ECG 5.5).

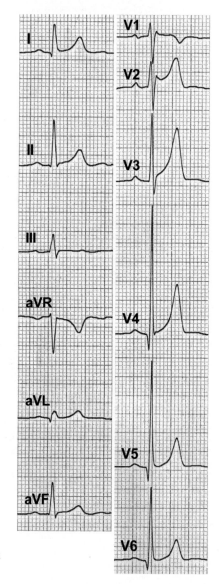

ECG 5.5 Electrocardiogram obtained from a 64-year-old man with mild aortic valve incompetence. Typical pattern of "diastolic overload." Relatively deep Q waves and tall, narrow R waves, slight ST elevation and positive, high, and peaked T waves in V_4 to V_6. The pattern is probably attributable to low rate sinus rhythm

For the diagnosis of common LVH in daily practice, we recommend the Cornell index (respecting the gender, see Table 5.2) and the Sokolow index (see Table 5.1) for high specificity. Unfortunately, the low sensitivity has to be accepted. However, the presence of strikingly high R waves in leads that are not represented by these two indices, or very deep S waves are present, LVH should be suspected (see the other indices in Table 5.1).

Diagnosis of Left Ventricular Hypertrophy in Intraventricular Conduction Disturbances

In the presence of left bundle-branch block (LBBB), and especially of left anterior fascicular block (LAFB), the diagnosis of LVH is markedly enhanced, for vectorial reasons. In contrast, the diagnosis is very much impaired in right bundle-branch block, because of partially opposite vectors of the left and right ventricle. In LBBB, the left ventricular vectors are unified in a single LV vector (see Chapter 10), thus improving the detection of LVH.

Based on the Framingham study, LVH is responsible for 70% of the cases of LBBB. Some indices have been published for the detection of LVH in LBBB. The index $S_{V1} + R_{V5}$ >45 mm of Klein et al. is simple, whereas the "index bundle" of Kafka et al. is complicated. Based on our own data, the specificity of Klein's index is good to excellent, but the sensitivity is significantly lower than that reported by these authors (ECG 5.6).

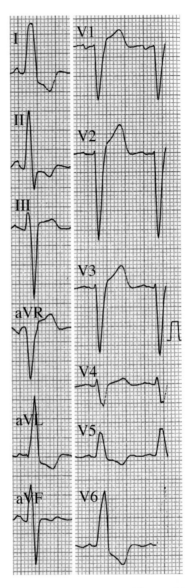

ECG 5.6 Electrocardiogram obtained from a 79-year-old man with left ventricular hypertrophy with left bundle-branch block, showing striking QRS amplitudes in the precordial leads (see calibration, $1\,mV = 5\,mm$). However, the index of Klein et al. ($S_{V1} + R_{V5} \geq 45\,mm$) is negative, at $42\,mm$

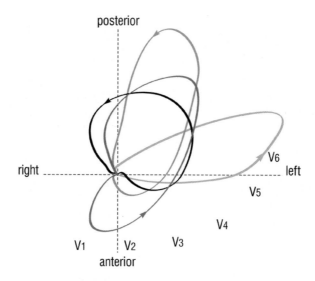

Figure 5.1 Variants of QRS vector loop (horizontal plane) in left anterior fascicular block

LAFB results in a unique, uniform behavior of the QRS complex in the frontal leads, a left axis deviation that facilitates the diagnosis of LVH. Moreover, the index mentioned below involves all variations of LV vectors in the horizontal plane (Figure 5.1). Consequently, the index $S_{III} + (R + S)_{maximal\ precordial} \geq 30$ mm (male) or ≥ 28 mm (female) is very reliable, with a specificity *and* sensitivity of 80%–90% (ECGs 5.7 and 5.8).

Right bundle-branch block reduces the R voltage in the lateral precordial leads (generally 2–5 mm) by RV vectors opposite to lateral LV vectors (see Chapter 10). Thus, LVH is probable if the amplitude of R waves in V_4 to V_6 is markedly greater than in a normal ECG (>12 mm). However, an echo is better by far.

The Short Story demonstrates a striking example of atypical LVH in a rare condition, hypertrophic obstructive cardiomyopathy (HOCM), in two young patients with completely different outcomes.

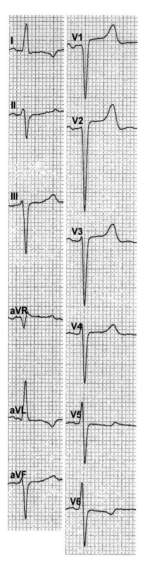

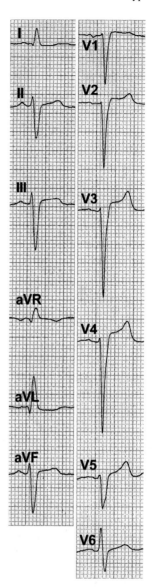

ECG 5.7 Electrocardiogram obtained from a 71-year-old man with left ventricular hypertrophy in left anterior fascicular block. The index $S_{III} + (R + S)_{maximal\ precordial} \geq 30\,mm$ is positive: $S_{III} = 12\,mm$; $R + S$ in $V_2 = 21\,mm$; sum $= 33\,mm$. All other voltage indices (e.g., R_{aVL}, $R_I + S_{III}$, Cornell, and Sokolow) are negative. Left ventricular mass $152\,g/m^2$

ECG 5.8 Electrocardiogram obtained from a 77-year-old man with left ventricular hypertrophy in left anterior fascicular block. Positive indices: Gertsch et al. (36 mm), Cornell (32 mm). Negative indices: R_{aVL}, $R_I + S_{III}$ and Sokolow. Left ventricular mass $160\,g/m^2$

Short Story/Case Report

On August 21, 1965, a 22-year-old man was investigated as the last patient in the ambulatory section of our department. He complained of anginal chest pain during strenuous exercise. He had a rough systolic murmur grade 3/6 over the fourth left intercostal space. X-rays showed the heart as slightly enlarged. His ECG was most spectacular (ECG 5.9a) and was first interpreted as an atypical pattern of a previous myocardial infarction. An instantaneous and intensive research in the literature, performed by all members of the department (only four at that time), revealed the probable presence of a recently described "new" cardiac disease, a "hypertrophic muscular subaortic stenosis," called hypertrophic obstructive cardiomyopathy (HOCM) today. Heart catheterization was planned for the next week.

The next morning, we investigated similar symptoms in a 27-year-old woman. She had the strange feeling that there was not enough room for the blood in her heart! Her ECG (ECG 5.9b) was so similar to that of the young man the evening before that we first thought of a mix-up between the two ECGs.

In both patients, the diagnosis of severe HOCM was confirmed by heart catheterization and left ventricular angiography, with an intraventricular gradient of 80 mmHg in each patient. We were confronted with an extremely rare duplicity of cases. However, the follow-up in these two young patients was completely different. The woman died suddenly 4 months later while playing tennis. Astonishingly, the man is still alive, 42 years later, without ever undergoing a heart operation and without heart failure, receiving minimal therapy (propranolol 40 mg a day) for more than 40 years. His hypertrophic obstructive cardiomyopathy converted over the decades into a nonobstructive modestly dilating cardiomyopathy.

The author never again encountered such extreme "HOCM-ECGs" in the following 42 years.

ECG 5.10 demonstrates an even rarer disease with LVH, apical hypertrophy. Note the enormous voltage of the R waves in the precordial leads combined with giant negative, symmetric T waves.

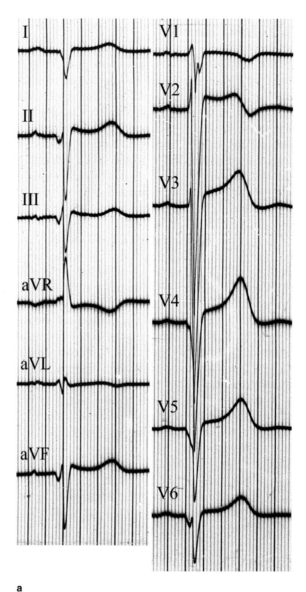

a

ECG 5.9 a. Electrocardiogram (ECG) obtained from a 22-year-old man with hypertrophic obstructive cardiomyopathy (HOCM) (see Short Story). ECG (50 mm/s): sinus rhythm (SR). Striking QRS vector in the limb and precordial leads. Frontal QRS axis ($\mathring{A}QRS_F$) approximately $-130°$, with a positive QRS complex only in lead aVR. Giant S waves in V_2/V_3. QS complexes in leads I, II, and V_4 to V_6

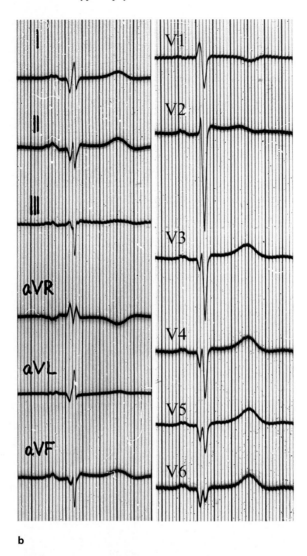

b

ECG 5.9 (continued) **b.** ECG from a 27-year-old woman with HOCM, also described in the Short Story. ECG (50 mm/s): SR. Striking QRS vector in the limb and precordial leads. ÅQRS$_F$ approximately −100°. QS complexes in leads V$_5$/V$_6$, prominent Q waves in leads I, II, aVL, aVF, and V$_3$/V$_4$. The QRS vector and the Q waves are very similar to those in part a

ECG 5.10 Electrocardiogram obtained from a 39-year-old man with apical hypertrophy. High R amplitude with significant ST depression and "giant," negative T waves in V_4 to V_6. Incomplete right bundle-branch block. Echo: left ventricular mass $270\,g/m^2$

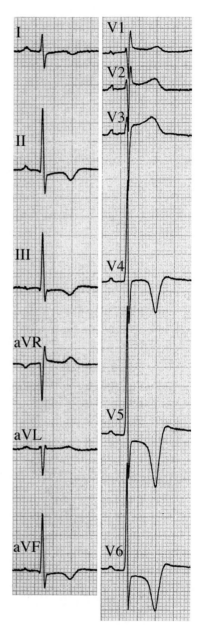

Chapter 6
Right Ventricular Hypertrophy

Right ventricular hypertrophy (RVH) is only detectable in the electrocardiogram (ECG) if the normally thin wall of the right ventricle (RV) develops hypertrophy up to a grade that more or less balances the left ventricular mass. This alteration always needs time, generally months or years.

Excessive RVH—an RV mass at least as great as the left ventricular mass—can be reliably diagnosed. In less severe RVH, the ECG manifestations allow only moderate suspicion for the presence of RVH. RVH is much rarer than left ventricular hypertrophy (LVH) and is encountered, in its extensive form, in several congenital heart diseases.

Etiology and Prevalence

Extensive RVH is observed in patients with congenital heart diseases such as Fallot's tetralogy, severe valvular pulmonary stenosis, and in the advanced stage of anomalies with left-to-right shunt complicated by Eisenmenger reaction. In acquired heart diseases such as cor pulmonale and mitral stenosis and after left heart failure, the ECG manifestations of RVH are in general quite moderate. Because of the limitations of the ECG in these cases, and in order to obtain further details, the echo is the method of choice. With echo, RVH can be quantified to a certain degree and RV function is measurable. Moderate to severe RVH is about 20 times rarer than LVH.

Lead V_1 is the most proximal to the anteriorly positioned right ventricle and therefore shows exclusively the direct and specific alterations of RVH, demonstrating the augmented RV vectors, directed anteriorly and to the right. Thus, lead V_1 represents the key lead for RVH, in the absence of a complete, or an incomplete, right bundle-branch block (RBBB). The special right precordial leads V_{3R} to V_{6R} are not used for the diagnosis or exclusion of RVH, but for the detection of acute RV infarction in the presence of acute inferior myocardial infarction.

M. Gertsch, *The ECG Manual: An Evidence-Based Approach,*
© Springer-Verlag London Limited 2009

Electrocardiogram Patterns in Right Ventricular Hypertrophy

RVH presents with three patterns: 1. without RV conduction disturbance, 2. with incomplete RBBB (iRBBB), and 3. with complete RBBB. Frontal QRS right axis deviation ($\text{Å}QRS_F \geq 90°$) is often present. Additional ST depression and especially T inversion in leads V_1 to V_2/V_3 favor the diagnosis of RVH in conditions 1 and 2, but not in 3.

Right Ventricular Hypertrophy Without Right Ventricular Conduction Disturbance

The ECG is characterized by a single positive QRS deflection in lead V_1 that is a pure R (ECGs 6.1 and 6.2). This condition is encountered in severe pulmonary valve stenosis (moderate forms can also be associated with iRBBB), severe RVH in congenital heart diseases with Eisenmenger syndrome, and, with a smaller R amplitude in V_1, in some cases of mitral stenosis and severe cor pulmonale. In general, there is associated $\text{Å}QRS_F$ deviation $>+120°$).

If some well-defined conditions, such as true posterior myocardial infarction and one type of preexcitation, are excluded, an R complex in V_1 is very specific for RVH. A qR complex in lead V_1 is a reliable sign of RV overload (ECG 6.3). The Q wave is attributable to RVH and right ventricular (and right atrial!) dilatation and not to anteroseptal necrosis. An RS complex in lead V_1 with an R/S ratio of more than 1:1 (ECG 6.4) favors the presence of RVH, but is less reliable. This is also valid for an R wave >7 mm in V_1 or an S wave <2 mm in V_1.

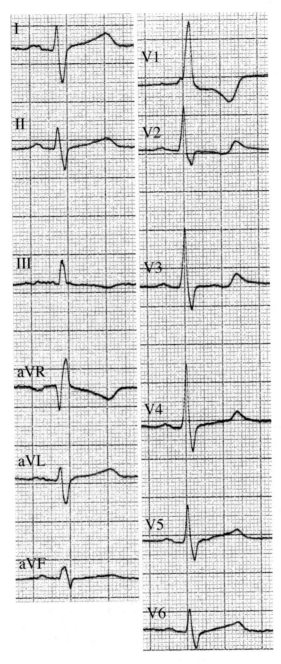

ECG 6.1 Electrocardiogram (ECG) obtained from a 19-year-old man with severe pulmonary valve stenosis (gradient 90 mmHg). ECG (paper speed 50 mm/s): frontal QRS axis +120°. Tall single R wave (15 mm), ST depression, and negative T wave in V_1. R > S in V_2 to V_4

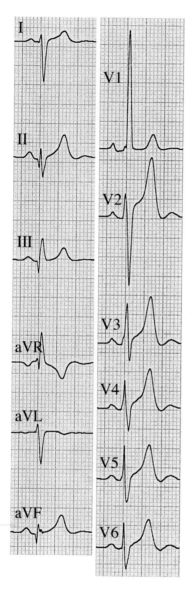

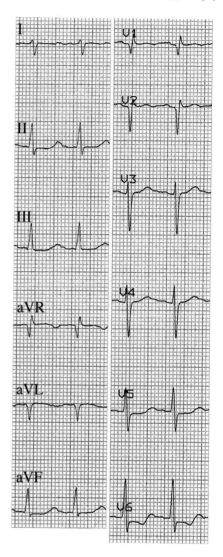

ECG 6.2 Electrocardiogram (ECG) obtained from a 27-year-old man with huge ventricular septal defect with early Eisenmenger REACTION at the age of 2 years. ECG: QRS right axis deviation. Single R wave (30 mm) in V_1. Positive T wave in all precordial leads

ECG 6.3 Electrocardiogram (ECG) obtained from a 43-year-old woman with severe mitral stenosis with tricuspid regurgitation. Mitral valve replacement and tricuspid De Vega plastique 2 years previously. ECG: sinus rhythm 116 beats/min. P duration >200 ms. The first peak of the p wave is partially hidden within the T wave. Atrioventricular block 1°. Frontal QRS axis +115°. Qr in V_1 and V_2. Alteration of the repolarization. Coro: normal

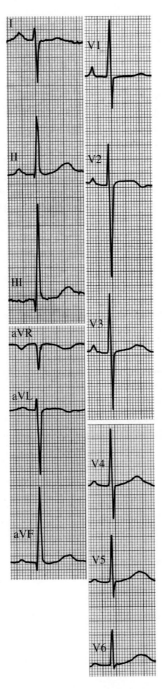

ECG 6.4 Electrocardiogram (ECG) obtained from a 2-year-old boy with Fallot's tetralogy, not operated. ECG (50 mm/s): QRS right axis deviation. R > S in lead V_1

Right Ventricular Hypertrophy with Incomplete Right Bundle-Branch Block (QRS Duration Normal)

An rSr′ complex in V_1 with an r′ smaller than the initial r wave is rarely associated with RVH and is rather common in healthy, young persons (ECG 6.5). If the r′ is obviously greater than the initial r wave, RVH is present in approximately 40% of the cases. On one hand, this rSr′ type (r′ > r) is typical for patients with an atrial septal defect of the secundum type (present in 90% in this anomaly), generally with asymmetric, negative T waves in V_1 to V_3 (ECG 6.6, where T negativity extends up to V_5) and may also be found in chronic pulmonary embolism, valvular pulmonary stenosis, and occasionally in cases with mitral stenosis. On the other hand, the pattern may occasionally represent an intermediate state between iRBBB and RBBB. The etiology in this case is manifold and includes fibrosis of the right bundle branch or coronary heart disease. However, it must be emphasized that an rSr′ type with r′ > r also occurs in normal individuals and is often found in patients with funnel chest.

Right Ventricular Hypertrophy with Complete Right Bundle-Branch Block (QRS Duration ≥0.12 s)

For RBBB with or without RVH, the typical pattern is an rsR′ complex in lead V_1. In some cases, the s wave is lacking because of projections and only a single broad and notched R wave is present. RVH can only be diagnosed or assumed, if the amplitude of R′ exceeds 12 mm, and/or the QRS duration is >0.14 s, caused by an atypically broad and often notched R′ wave. An associated frontal QRS right axis between +80° and +120° is required (ECG 6.7). The T wave is always negative in lead V_1, in many cases also in V_2 to V_4, with and without RVH.

In all cases of RVH, the classical pattern of associated right atrial hypertrophy, the "p pulmonale," can only be detected in patients with cor pulmonale "parenchymal," because of obstructive lung disease. Statistically, RBBB is much more frequent in patients without RVH than with it (at about 20:1). It is advisable to correlate the ECG with the clinical findings, especially in borderline "ECG RVH," and to use the echo as a direct and better diagnostic method.

Rare Right Ventricular Hypertrophy Patterns

An $S_I/S_{II}/S_{III}$ pattern can indicate RVH in some instances but is more often found in normal individuals. In rare cases, RVH manifests in a negative QRS complex in all precordial leads, with or without iRBBB; in the frontal plane, there is often QRS right axis deviation. ECG 6.8 shows an example of an (r)Sr′s′ complex in V_1.

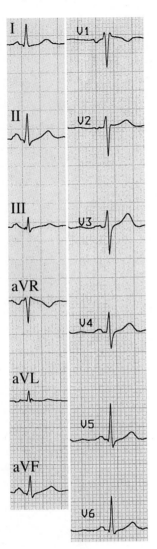

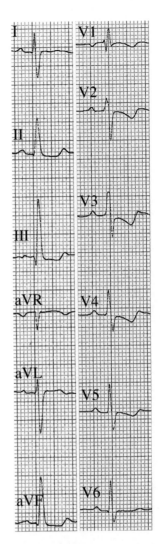

ECG 6.5 Electrocardiogram (ECG) obtained from a 51-year-old woman with a normal heart. ECG: incomplete right bundle-branch block with r′ < r, as a normal variant.

ECG 6.6 Electrocardiogram (ECG) obtained from a 49-year-old woman with atrial septal defect of the secundum type, left to right shunt >60%. Pulmonary artery pressure normal. ECG: frontal QRS axis +105°. Incomplete right bundle-branch block with r′ > r, T negative up to lead V$_5$

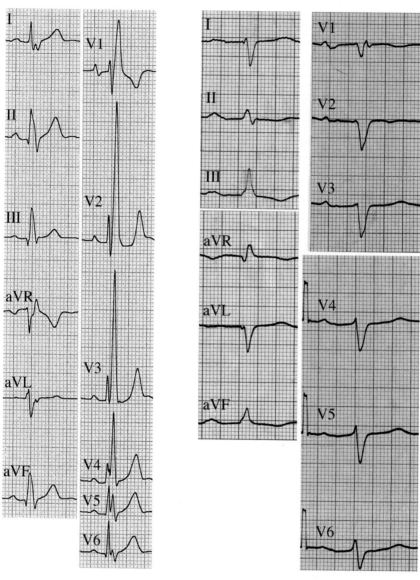

ECG 6.7 Electrocardiogram (ECG) obtained from a 26-year-old man with Fallot's tetralogy operated 10 years previously. ECG: frontal QRS axis (of the first 60 ms) +75°. Direct pattern of right bundle-branch block in V_1 up to V_5 (V_6), with giant amplitude of R' in V_2/V_3, corresponding to persisting severe right ventricular hypertrophy confirmed with the echo

ECG 6.8 Electrocardiogram (ECG) obtained from a 73-year-old woman with chronic obstructive pulmonary disease with global respiratory failure. Hypertension and pulmonary arterial hypertension. Right ventricular heart failure. ECG (50 mm/s): sinus rhythm. Frontal QRS axis +110°. rS complex in all precordial leads. Thorax x-rays: Cor bovinum. No echo. This rare pattern may also be seen in smaller hearts

Chapter 7
Biventricular Hypertrophy

Reliable detection of biventricular hypertrophy (BVH) is accomplished with the echocardiogram. With the electrocardiogram (ECG), the diagnosis can only be made if excessive right ventricular hypertrophy (RVH) preponderates left ventricular hypertrophy (LVH).

The following "classical" ECG configuration is proposed for the diagnosis of BVH:

1. $S_{V1} + R_{V5(or\ V6)}$ <35 mm (positive Sokolow index), combined with frontal QRS right axis deviation ($\mathring{A}QRS_F \geq +90°$). The index can only be used in patients 30 years or older. It has an acceptable specificity of approximately 70%–80% but an extremely low sensitivity.
2. $S_{V6} \geq 7$ mm (without right bundle-branch block). This sign is also seen in isolated RVH.
3. Probably the best sign for BVH is the combination of some typical RVH patterns with left atrial (LA) enlargement (p duration ≥120 ms).

    a. S/R ≥1 in V_5/V_6 + LA enlargement
    b. $S_{V6} \geq 7$ mm + LA enlargement (ECG 7.1)
    c. $\mathring{A}QRS_F > +90°$ + LA enlargement (in the presence of right bundle-branch block, the $\mathring{A}QRS_F$ is determined on the basis of the first 60 ms of QRS)

The above three criteria have a good specificity (approximately 80%) but a very low sensitivity. Another ECG sign is a striking discrepancy between a shallow S wave in V_1 and a deep S wave in V_2 (shallow S_{V1}/deep S_{V2} sign; see ECG 7.2). The right ventricular vector partially cancels the left ventricular vector in lead V_1, but has little influence on lead V_2, because of projection. Again, the specificity is quite good and the sensitivity low. The sign can be false positive if lead V_1 is placed too high and/or too far right laterally.

In suspected cases of BVH, an echocardiogram and other diagnostics such as heart catheterization and investigations for lung diseases are necessary to identify the disease(s) that lead to BVH.

M. Gertsch, *The ECG Manual: An Evidence-Based Approach*,   67
© Springer-Verlag London Limited 2009

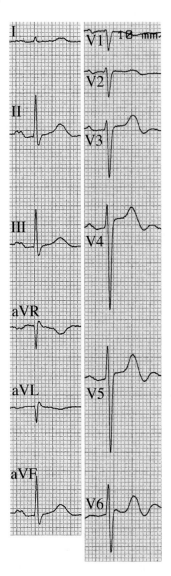

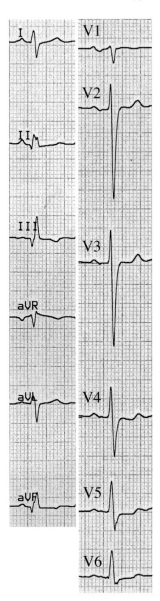

ECG 7.1 Electrocardiogram (ECG) obtained from an 83-year-old woman. S_{V_6} >7 mm and left atrial (LA) enlargement. Combined aortic valve disease, severe mitral regurgitation. ECG: sinus rhythm. p Duration 120 ms: S in V_6 10 mm. The rS configuration in V_1 to V_6 suggests right ventricular and/or left ventricular dilatation. Echo: hypertrophic and dilated right and left ventricle. Dilated atria. Thoracic x-rays: cor bovinum

ECG 7.2 Electrocardiogram obtained from a 73-year-old man. "Shallow S_{V_1}/deep S_{V_2}." Combined aortic and mitral valve disease. Sinus rhythm, p duration 120 ms. Frontal QRS axis +110°. S_{V_1} = 3.5 mm, S_{V_2} = 14 mm. Negative T waves in V_1 to V_4. Echo: biventricular hypertrophy and dilatation

Chapter 8
Pulmonary Embolism

Acute pulmonary embolism (acPE), limited to the first 48 hours of the disease, is a very dangerous situation with considerable mortality, often as a result of misdiagnosis. It is therefore necessary to establish the diagnosis and to begin therapy in the shortest possible time. The fastest and most reliable methods are the echocardiogram and helical (spiral) computed tomography, combined with plasma D-dimer measurement. With this approach, diagnostic accuracy is approximately 95%, and pulmonary artery angiography can be avoided in most cases.

A positive result from lower limb venous compression ultrasonography is useful for the diagnosis, especially in subacute pulmonary embolism (subacPE), with symptoms lasting for >48 hours. Lung scan is only diagnostic in approximately 50% of cases, but is helpful for the diagnosis of subsegmental embolization. On one hand, the electrocardiogram (ECG) is unreliable for the diagnosis of acPE; on the other hand, it may represent the first indication of right ventricular (RV) overload.

Acute and Subacute Pulmonary Embolism

The arbitrary differentiation between acPE (first 48 hours after the event) and subacPE (symptoms lasting longer than 2 days) is not particularly helpful in daily practice because the beginning of the disease is not precisely determinable in each case. Moreover, there are no significant differences in the ECG between acPE and subacPE. Chronic pulmonary embolization, lasting weeks, months, or even years, is discussed at the end of the chapter.

In acPE and subacPE, the more or less *acute* rise of pulmonary artery resistance leads to dilatation (not to hypertrophy) of the right ventricle and of the right atrium, because of acute right heart failure. Pulmonary arterial pressure often increases only modestly. As a consequence, the following ECG alterations may be present.

M. Gertsch, *The ECG Manual: An Evidence-Based Approach*,
© Springer-Verlag London Limited 2009

Alterations of QRS

1. Shift of the frontal QRS axis to the right, often with a S_I/Q_{III} (condition: $S_I \geq 1.5$ mm; $Q_{III} \geq 1.5$ mm) or S_I/rSr'_{III}.
2. Rotation of the heart in its horizontal axis (also provoked by RV dilatation), leading to clockwise displacement of the transition zone (= QRS clockwise rotation) in the precordial leads. If QRS counterclockwise rotation is encountered, it is the result of preexisting RV hypertrophy or other causes.
3. RV conduction disturbance: incomplete (or rarely complete) right bundle-branch block (RBBB), with rSr' complex (or rsR' complex in complete RBBB) in lead V_1.

A QR complex (Qr) in lead V_1 is seen in approximately 10% of cases, especially in massive pulmonary embolism (>80% obstruction of the pulmonary arteries).

Alterations of Repolarization

a. T negativity in III *and* aVF.
b. T negativity in V_2/V_3, also without incomplete RBBB or RBBB.
c. ST depression in leads V_1 to V_3, or ST elevation in leads V_1 and III.
d. ST or T alterations in the left precordial leads (rare).

Rhythm Disturbances

Sinus tachycardia is by far the most frequent ECG abnormality in acPE, in 70%–90% of cases. Atrial flutter occurs in 5%–10%, whereas atrial fibrillation is rare.

Alterations of the p Wave

Relatively high and peaked p waves may be seen in some leads, especially in II and V_2. The definition of this alteration (also described as *p pulmonale vasculare*) is a conundrum and so is its prevalence. The classical "p pulmonale" ("p pulmonale parenchymal" with an amplitude ≥ 2.5 mm in lead II, and purely negative in aVL) is seen only exceptionally. Possible ECG signs in acPE are listed in Table 8.1.

It needs to be emphasized that eventual ECG signs attributed to acPE are transitory and reversible in successfully treated patients. The existence of several, different ECG signs of ventricular overload is helpful, although still insufficient, for the diagnosis of acPE. ECGs 8.1–8.4 were registered in patients with massive acPE at admission to the emergency unit of our hospital during the winter of 2001. AcPE was proven by helical computed tomography (and echocardiography).

Table 8.1 Possible ECG signs in acPE (based on the literature)

	Prevalence (%)
1. Sinus tachycardia (rate ≥100 beats/min)	70
Sinus rhythm (rate ≥90%)	80
2. S_I/Q_{III} type or S_I/rSr'_{III} type	40
3. S_I/Q_{III} *or* S_I/rSr'_{III} + negative T in III and aVF	25
4. Incomplete RSB (rSr' or QR in V_1) 40%	7(!)–60
5. QRS clockwise rotation in precordial leads	35
6. ÅQRS$_F$ shift to the right up to ≥+60° at the age >30 years	30
7. T negativity in leads V_2 and V_3	30
8. Right atrial enlargement (atypical "p pulmonale")	10?
9. Atrial flutter	5
10. Complete RBBB	3

ECG, electrocardiogram; ÅQRS$_F$, frontal QRS axis; acPE, acute pulmonary embolism; RBBB, right bundle-branch block.

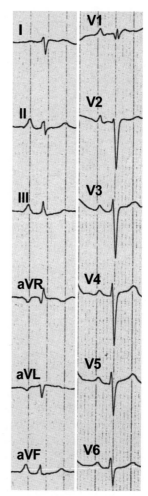

ECG 8.1 Electrocardiogram obtained from a 53-year-old woman. Sinus rhythm 93 beats/min. Peaked p waves inferiorly and in V_1/V_3 (rare finding). Frontal QRS axis +140°, peripheral QRS low voltage. S_I, but no Q_{III}. Incomplete right bundle-branch block. Excessive clockwise rotation in the precordial leads, rS up to V_6. No negative T waves in the right or other precordial leads. Five possible signs of acute right ventricular overload

ECG 8.2 Electrocardiogram obtained from a 34-year-old woman. Sinus tachycardia 104 beats/min. Negative p wave in V_1 as a sign of left atrial overload. Frontal QRS axis +75°. S_I/Q_{III} type. Incomplete right bundle-branch block with Qr in V_1. Clockwise rotation. Slight ST elevation in V_1 (and V_2/V_3). ST depression in V_5/V_6. No negative T waves. Five signs

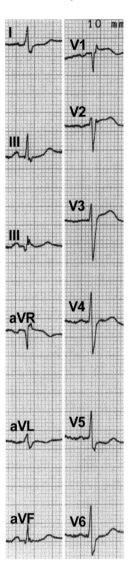

Only two of the four patients showed five current ECG signs of RV overload and another showed only one or two signs. Three patients had sinus tachycardia. Three patients recovered with thrombolysis, whereas a 34-year-old woman (ECG 8.2) admitted 2 weeks after a delivery died despite thrombolysis and surgical thrombectomy.

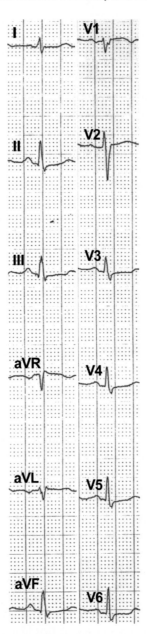

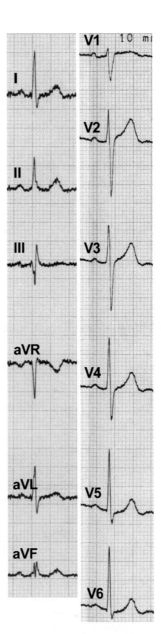

ECG 8.3 Electrocardiogram obtained from a 43-year-old woman. Sinus rhythm 92 beats/min; normal p. Frontal QRS axis +80°. S_I/Q_{III} type. Pseudo-incomplete right bundle-branch block. No clockwise rotation, no T negativity in precordial leads. Two signs

ECG 8.4 Electrocardiogram obtained from a 53-year-old woman. Sinus rhythm 79 beats/min; normal p. Frontal QRS axis approximately +40°. S_I/rSr'_{III} type. Slight clockwise rotation. No T negativity. One sign

The following are some general comments on the findings in ECGs 8.1–8.4:

1. All patients in this group were women. However, the ratio of female to male in acPE is approximately 3:2.
2. All patients had massive life-threatening acPE with corresponding symptoms (tachypnea, severe dyspnea at rest, hemoptysis in two cases) and clinical findings (preshock, distended jugular veins, cyanosis and sinus tachycardia in three cases).

These examples and the literature support the general opinion that the ECG is unreliable for diagnosis of acPE, because of its modest specificity and low sensitivity. Therefore, it should not be used as a diagnostic method. In many patients, preexisting ECG alterations may be falsely suggestive for acPE and, much worse, the ECG may lack any sign of RV overload even in patients with massive acPE. Moreover, it is often impossible to differentiate between signs of RV overload and normal variants (see Chapter 3).

The Value of the Electrocardiogram

If the ECG is unreliable for the diagnosis of PE, where then is the place for the ECG in suspected acPE?

1. *Differentiation of acute myocardial infarction (AMI) from acPE.*
   As every physician knows, the diagnosis of acPE based on symptoms (and anamnestic findings) is not always easy to make. Often, AMI has to be excluded. Generally, in inferior AMI, a striking ST elevation is seen in leads III, aVF, and II. An older inferior infarction shows not only pathologic Q waves in III and aVF, but also a Q (q) wave in II. In contrast, a Q (q) wave in lead II is extremely rare in acute RV overload. AMI of other localization may be detected by the usual criteria.
2. *Analysis of heart rhythm and conduction disturbances.*
   Arrhythmias and conduction disturbances can only be reliably diagnosed with the ECG.
3. *In the presence of ECG signs suggesting acute RV overload, the diagnosis of acPE (or subacPE) should be confirmed or excluded as soon as possible.*
   Patients with acPE, and especially with subacPE, may have a conundrum history and puzzling symptoms. We have observed a substantial number of patients whose multiple ECG signs of RV overload have represented the first hint for the diagnosis of pulmonary embolism. This has occurred more often in subacPE than in acPE. It is important to note that only a minority of the hospitals worldwide have a spiral computed tomograph and an experienced specialist in echo/Doppler available at any given time. In these circumstances, the ECG may be helpful for the diagnosis of acPE, together with the history, symptoms, and other clinical findings.

The regression of ECG signs of RV overload, if present in acPE or subacPE, may be a useful indicator of a favorable clinical follow up. However, there is no strict time correlation between the objective findings (e.g., in the echo) and the ECG. The alterations may regress sooner or persist longer than expected.

The Short Story describes a patient whose life was saved by timely and prompt action.

Short Story/Case Report

On October 11, 2000, a 61-year-old man was admitted to the emergency department of our hospital because of sudden onset of severe dyspnea and syncope 3 hours before. Rapid clinical examination revealed a life-threatening condition evidenced by shock (systolic blood pressure 70/40 mmHg, heart rate 135 beats/min), breathing frequency of 50/min, cyanosis, and thick neck veins. The patient was not able to give further information. An emergency transthoracic echocardiography revealed severe RV and right atrial dilatation. The left ventricle showed subnormal contraction. The ECG (ECG 8.5) was interpreted as suspicious for acute RV overload. However, the lacking Q in III and a QR complex in V_1 as well as a QS complex in V_2, together with slight ST elevation, led to momentary confusion (anteroseptal AMI?). Fifteen minutes after admission, echocardiographically confirmed electromechanical dissociation with ventricular asystole occurred, thus instantaneously vigorous cardiopulmonary resuscitation (CPR) was performed. At the same time, two intravenous bolus injections of 15 mg of alteplase were given, followed by infusion of 70 mg within 60 minutes, whereby CPR was continued. Twenty-five minutes later, spontaneous carotid pulses were observed, and the patient's hemodynamics recovered with support of catecholamines. Emergency spiral computed tomography revealed a >80% occlusion of the proximal pulmonary arteries. The patient was transferred to the intensive care unit. Three hours after successful CPR and thrombolysis, the patient developed hemorrhagic shock because of liver and spleen rupture as a consequence of prolonged mechanical chest compression and abdominal blood pooling caused by severely impaired RV function. After emergency splenectomy and liver revision, the patient's hemodynamics stabilized 14 hours after admission. Ten days after successful treatment of acute central PE, there were no signs of RV overload as shown by normalization of the echocardiogram and the ECG.

This patient's life was saved because, based on typical clinical symptoms, echo, and ECG findings, strongly suggesting massive acPE, instantaneous resuscitation and rapid thrombolysis were applied. The patient was fortunate to survive a further, severe complication. The basic disease for the development of thrombosis of deep lower limb veins, without symptoms, remained unclear. The retrospective detailed analysis of the ECG on admission revealed, besides sinus tachycardia, at least six signs of acute RV overload (ECG 8.5). The QR and QS complexes in V_1/V_2, together with slight ST elevation, proved to be ominous

ECG 8.5 Electrocardiogram (ECG) obtained from a 60-year-old man described in the Short Story. ECG: sinus tachycardia 120 beats/min. Peaked p waves in II/aVF. Frontal QRS axis +100°. S_I/Rs_{III} type (in this case equivalent to S_I/Q_{III} type, because of extreme rotation of the heart). Qr complex in V_1 (and QS complex in V_2). Clockwise rotation in precordial leads. ST elevation of 0.5–1.0 mm in V_1/V_2. T negativity in V_2. At least seven signs

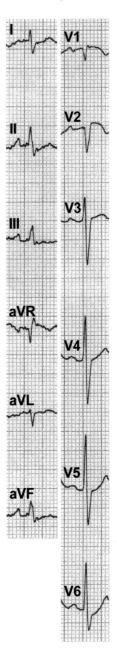

signs of extreme RV and right atrial dilatation and were not the result of anteroseptal AMI.

Chronic, Repetitive Pulmonary Embolism

In chronic, repetitive PE, RV hypertrophy develops. Significant pulmonary hypertension is present, combined with right heart failure, sometimes of modest degree. The ECG may or may not reveal RV hypertrophy. The correct diagnosis is often overlooked.

Chapter 9
Fascicular Blocks

The concept of fascicular blocks is based on the predominantly trifascicular infrahisian ventricular conduction system, the right bundle branch on one side and the left anterior and left posterior fascicle forming the left bundle branch on the other side (Figure 9.1). The expression *fascicular block* is synonymous with the older expression *hemiblock*. This is reasonable because, in approximately 10% of the human intraventricular conduction system, there is a third left ventricular fascicle called *medial fascicle* of a plurifascicular system, and this impairs diagnostic accuracy.

Generally, the lesion responsible for the block is localized very proximally in the fascicle, near the His bundle. Rarely, in some individuals, fascicular blocks progress to bifascicular/bilateral blocks: right bundle-branch block (RBBB) + left anterior fascicular block (LAFB) or RBBB + left posterior fascicular block (LPFB) (see Chapter 11) and then to complete atrioventricular block (see Chapter 12). Thus, fascicular blocks represent potential precursors of infrahisian complete atrioventricular block, which is often associated with syncope and premature, sudden death.

Etiology and Prevalence

LAFB and LPFB are both left (mono-) fascicular blocks but differ greatly in prevalence and etiology and in correct diagnosis. The etiology of isolated LAFB is manifold, including left ventricular hypertrophy (LVH), coronary heart disease with or without myocardial infarction, fibrosis of the infrahisian conduction system (Lenègre's disease), and others. Isolated LPFB is the result of inferior myocardial infarction in about 90% of the cases. In the general population, LAFB develops after the age of 40 years, is found in 4%–6% of those aged 60 and older, and 10% of those aged 80 years. Rarely, LAFB completely masks an inferior or anterior infarction.

LPFB is rare in middle-aged patients seen in a medical or cardiology department (0.15% and 0.3%, respectively) and is even rarer in a general population. The reason is a relative great caliber of the left posterior fascicle, an early and separate ramification from the His bundle, and a double blood supply. However, the diagnosis is important because LPFB is combined with inferior myocardial infarction in most

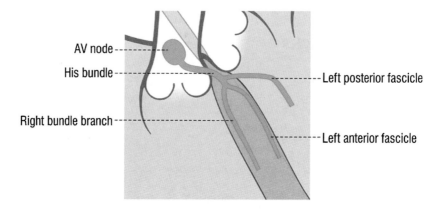

Figure 9.1 Trifascicular ventricular conduction system

cases. In inferior infarction, LPFB is found in 6% of cases, and often masks the classical infarction signs. If we assume a mean normal QRS duration of 0.09 s, the QRS duration in LAFB and in LPFB is prolonged to 0.10–0.11 s, without LVH.

Left Anterior Fascicular Block

LAFB is easy to diagnose. The first main characteristic of LAFB is a QRS left axis deviation in the frontal leads, with a frontal QRS axis (ÅQRS$_F$) between −30° and −90°. Leads I and aVL produce a single R wave; a small q wave in these leads may be present but an s wave is rare. In leads I and aVL, a slurred R downstroke is often found. In the inferior leads II, aVF, and III there is an rS complex. The T wave is positive and asymmetric in these leads, negative in aVR, and positive, flat, or negative in I and aVL (ECG 9.1).

The second main characteristic of LAFB, which is often forgotten in the literature, is a smooth transition zone of QRS in the horizontal leads with an RS configuration in all precordial leads (ECG 9.1). Generally, there is an rS complex (s smaller than R) in V$_1$ to V$_6$. In some cases, R and S have approximately the same amplitude in V$_2$/V$_3$ and/or V$_4$ to V$_6$, and very rarely R is higher than S in V$_2$/V$_3$ or V$_5$/V$_6$ (ECG 9.2). This electrocardiogram (ECG) produces a small s wave in I and the mirror image of the slurred R wave in III. In LAFB, the T wave is positive and asymmetric in all precordial leads. In rare cases, there is a small q wave in V$_1$ and V$_2$ (qrS), which more frequently represents a normal variant of LAFB than an anteroseptal infarction (ECG 9.3). The small q wave present here in V$_3$ to V$_6$ is very rare.

Note that the left axis deviation (ÅQRS$_F$ between −30° and −90°) is attributable to LAFB in approximately 90% of cases; in 10%, other conditions are responsible for this abnormality: inferior infarction (5%) and rare conditions such as LVH, thoracic anomalies, and others (5%). However, in these cases, we always miss a slurred R downstroke in leads I and aVL and a smooth transition zone in the precordial leads.

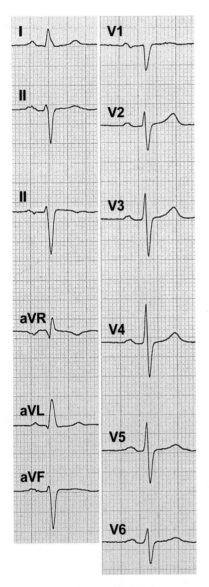

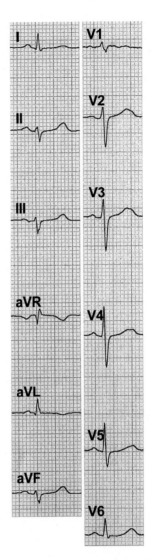

ECG 9.1 Electrocardiogram obtained from a 74-year-old man with typical left anterior fascicular block. Frontal QRS axis −75°, slurred R downstroke in I/aVL, and "smooth" transition zone in precordial leads

ECG 9.2 Electrocardiogram obtained from a 54-year-old man with typical left anterior fascicular block. Frontal QRS axis −60°, mirror image of slurred R downstroke in III, and smooth transition zone in precordial leads. $R < S$ in V_5/V_6

ECG 9.3 Electrocardiogram obtained from a 52-year-old man with variant of left anterior fascicular block, with small Q waves in leads V_2 and V_3 (V_4). As usual, no Q wave in V_6. Differential diagnosis: previous anteroseptal myocardial infarction

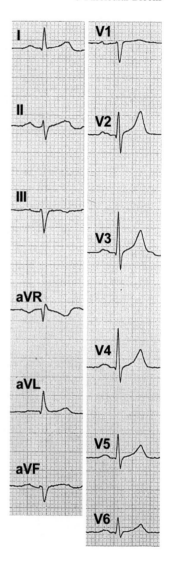

Left Posterior Fascicular Block

LPFB is difficult to diagnose because only minor alterations may allow the differentiation from a normal variant with vertical ÅQRS$_F$. LPFB is frequently associated with inferior infarction and, in this condition, is characterized by a ÅQRS$_F$ between +50° and +80°, by a q wave of variable duration in III and aVF, and variable T waves in the same leads. Generally, there is a slurred R downstroke in leads III and aVF. The alterations in the precordial leads are minimal but of diagnostic value. In most cases, we also find a slurred R downstroke in V_6, and there is no s wave (ECG 9.4) or only a minimal s wave in this lead.

ECG 9.4 Electrocardiogram obtained from a 68-year-old man with left posterior fascicular block, partly masking previous inferior myocardial infarction. Frontal QRS axis +55°. Q wave <0.04 s in III and aVF. Slurred R downstroke in II (III/aVF) and V_6/V_5. Negative T wave in III. Note the absence of S wave in V_6 (and V_5). Coro: closed right coronary artery, inferior aneurysm, ejection fraction 42%

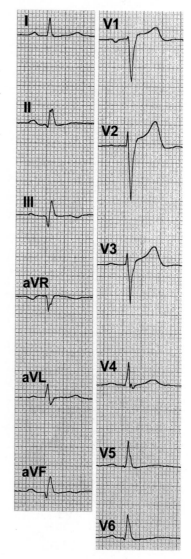

LPFB masks the pattern of previous inferior infarction partially or completely. The difference between the ECG pattern of previous inferior myocardial infarction without LPFB and that associated with LPFB is obvious. Instead of the typical loss of QRS vectors resulting in pathologic Q waves (≥0.04 s) or QS waves in leads III and aVF (II), often with negative and symmetric T waves (ECG 9.5), we find tall R waves with small or only slightly enlarged or absent Q waves, combined with negative, flat, or positive T waves (ECGs 9.4 and 9.6). The extremely rare LPFB without inferior infarction shows the aforementioned pattern with small q waves and even greater R waves in the inferior leads, leading to a $\mathring{A}QRS_F$ between +80° and +120°.

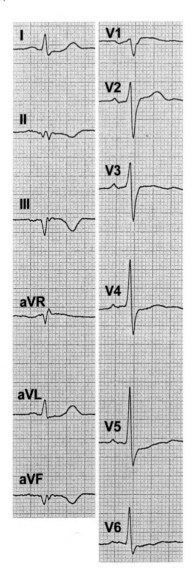

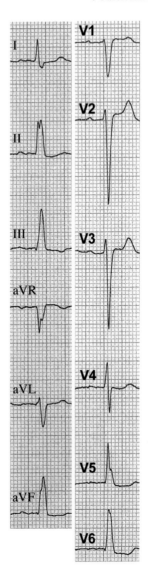

ECG 9.5 Electrocardiogram obtained from a 73-year-old man with previous inferior myocardial infarction without left posterior fascicular block. Frontal QRS axis −50°. Q > 0.04 s in III and aVF (II), and symmetric negative T waves in the same leads

ECG 9.6 Electrocardiogram obtained from a 72-year-old woman with left posterior fascicular block, completely masking previous inferior myocardial infarction. Left atrial enlargement. Frontal QRS axis +80°. Slurred R downstroke in V_5 and as mirror image in aVR. Tall and broad R waves in II, aVF, and III. Only minimal Q waves in the same leads. Coro: closed right coronary artery, inferior akinesia, ejection fraction 50%

The pattern of LPFB in its common combination with inferior infarction can easily be confounded with other conditions with an $\mathring{A}QRS_F$ between +50° and +80° or even +120°, for example, a normal ECG in young individuals (especially with asthenic habitus) (ECG 9.7) or in patients with right ventricular hypertrophy. For the correct diagnosis, the QRS duration, the fine alterations described above (especially in lead V6), and a history of inferior myocardial infarction must be considered. In doubtful cases, an inferior infarction can be confirmed or excluded by echocardiography.

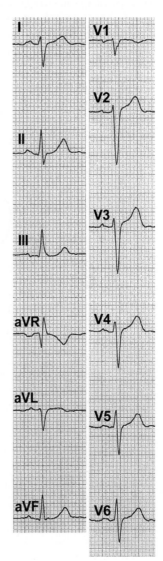

ECG 9.7 Electrocardiogram obtained from a 32-year-old man with no apparent heart disease, weight 115 kg. Unclear right axis deviation. Frontal QRS axis approximately +130°. No signs for left posterior fascicular block (note also broad S wave in V_6 and small S wave in aVF)

Diagnosis of Left Ventricular Hypertrophy
in Left Anterior Fascicular Block

Astonishingly, the detection of LVH is markedly improved in LAFB, for vectorial reasons. In the ECG with normal conduction and especially with RBBB, the direction of the left and right ventricular vectors is partially opposed, making the construction of a reasonable index impossible. Moreover, the ÅQRS_F is extremely variable in these conditions, but somewhat less so in LBBB.

In contrast, in LAFB, the ÅQRS_F is per definition a left axis deviation and by the behavior of the horizontal part of the QRS complex, all variations of the R + S complex can be validated (Figure 9.2). Thus, with the index for LVH in LAFB, S_{III} + (R + S)$_{\text{maximal precordial}}$ may be improved to 80%–90%, for specificity *and* sensitivity (see Chapter 5, ECGs 5.7 and 5.8).

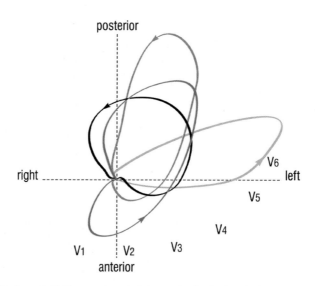

Figure 9.2 Horizontal QRS vector loop in left anterior fascicular block

Chapter 10
Complete and Incomplete Bundle-Branch Blocks

Bundle-branch blocks are the most common electrocardiogram (ECG) patterns of aberration of the ventricular conduction, in the presence of a supraventricular rhythm, mostly sinus rhythm. This means that the electric impulse is conducted through one bundle branch and blocked in the other. Consequently, one ventricle is activated normally and the other with delay through the interventricular septum.

Other types of aberration in the ventricles are fascicular blocks (including bifascicular and/or bilateral blocks) and preexcitation in individuals with an accessory pathway. For any physician, the differentiation between complete right bundle-branch block (RBBB) and complete left bundle-branch block (LBBB) is almost as important as the differentiation between right-hand drive and left-hand drive for the general population.

The prevalence of RBBB depends predominantly on age and the presence or absence of coronary heart disease. Overall, RBBB seems to be more frequent than LBBB. The etiologies for both blocks are, among others, hypertension, coronary heart disease, degenerative disease of the intraventricular conduction system (Lenègre's disease), and heart valve replacement.

The normal human ECG is a "levogram" because of the important muscle mass of the left ventricle (LV) compared with that of the right ventricle (RV), at a ratio of 8:1. Thus, the great LV vectors outweigh the small RV vectors. In the 12-lead ECG, we generally do not see anything of the RV excitation, with two exceptions: RV hypertrophy (RVH) (see Chapter 6) and RBBB.

The expression *conduction block* may be misleading. Often, there is no real conduction block but an extensive slowing of the conduction. This explains why the block may be incomplete or complete. Also, in complete blocks, an extreme reduction of the conduction velocity may be the reason for the pattern of bundle-branch block. Moreover, the block may be reversible, for example, after heart operation, after recovery from myocardial infarction, pulmonary embolism (RBBB), or infectious heart disease, in some cases after thoracic trauma (RBBB), or by treatment of arterial hypertension (mostly LBBB).

M. Gertsch, *The ECG Manual: An Evidence-Based Approach*,
© Springer-Verlag London Limited 2009

Complete Right Bundle-Branch Block

RBBB and LBBB are characterized by a broad QRS complex and a special QRS configuration. QRS duration in LBBB is generally longer than in RBBB. Without concomitant ventricular hypertrophy, QRS in RBBB measures 0.12–0.14 s and in LBBB 0.14–0.16 s, rarely only 0.12 s. QRS duration is generally longer in LBBB than in RBBB, because the completely abnormal excitation of the septum and the free wall of the LV in LBBB takes more time.

In RBBB, RV excitation is exceptionally detectable, because the RV is activated *after* the LV. The activation of the LV and RV can be seen separately. The QRS vector in RBBB is similar to that of normal ventricular activation, with the exception of the last part. The initial and middle vectors are only slightly altered, whereas the delayed excitation of the RV produces a great vector oriented to the right (Figures 10.1 and 10.2). There are only two leads in the 12-lead standard ECG that explore rightward-oriented vectors directly, which is by a positive deflection: V_1 and aVR, and, to a certain degree, lead III. For RBBB, a terminal broad R wave is characteristic in these leads. In lead V_1, the classical pattern is an rsR′ complex with an R′ of great amplitude, approximately 5–16 mm (ECG 10.1). In some cases, a simple broad but always notched R complex is present, because of projections (ECG 10.2). If an RSR′ complex is present in V_1 to V_3 (V_4), RVH must be suspected, especially if a frontal QRS axis $\geq +90°$ is found.

In uncomplicated RBBB, a qR type in V_1 is rare and RVH must be excluded in this case. The positive terminal R wave in aVR and often also in III confirms the diagnosis of RBBB. The absence of a terminal R wave in aVR excludes RBBB, and other conditions for a single R wave in lead V_1 such as preexcitation or posterior myocardial infarction must be considered. A qR type is seen also in RBBB associated with anteroseptal infarction. In RBBB, leads I, aVL, and V_5/V_6, as mirror image leads for the delayed RV activation, show broad terminal S waves with an amplitude of 1–6 mm.

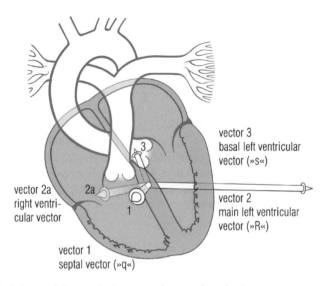

Figure 10.1 Scheme of the ventricular vectors in normal conduction

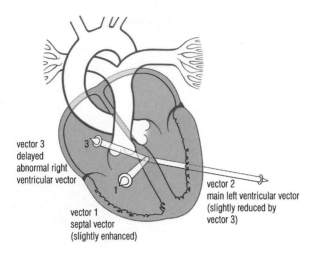

vector 3
delayed
abnormal right
ventricular vector

3

1

vector 1
septal vector
(slightly enhanced)

vector 2
main left ventricular vector
(slightly reduced by
vector 3)

Figure 10.2 Scheme of the ventricular vectors in right bundle-branch block

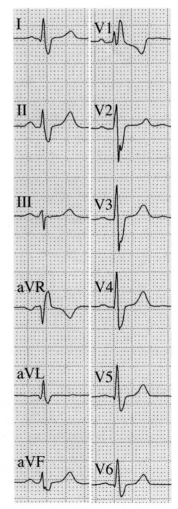

ECG 10.1 Electrocardiogram obtained from a 33-year-old man. Right bundle-branch block with the typical RSR′ (rsR′) configuration only in V_1. Normal heart

ECG 10.2 Electrocardiogram obtained from a
58-year-old woman. Right bundle-branch block without
an rsR′ complex in V_1, but with a notched broad
R wave in V_1/V_2 and an Rsr′ complex in V_3.
Hypertension, normal heart

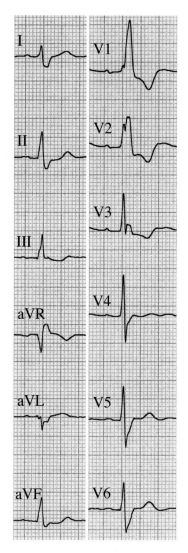

Incomplete Right Bundle-Branch Block

Incomplete RBBB (iRBBB) is characterized by an rSr′ complex in lead V_1, always
with a terminal r wave in lead aVR. The r′ wave in V_1 may be smaller, equal, or
greater than the initial r wave. Generally, the pattern is common (up to 5%) and is
considered a normal variant in most cases (ECG 10.3). An r′ wave in V_1 significantly broader than the initial r wave may be caused by RVH or enlargement,
especially if the T waves are negative in V_2 and V_3 or up to $V_{4/5}$ (ECG 10.4).

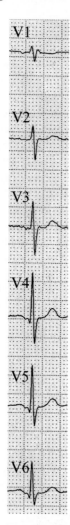

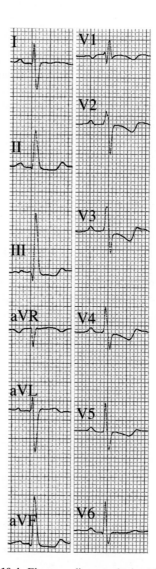

ECG 10.3 Electrocardiogram obtained from a 31-year-old man. Incomplete right bundle-branch block with r > r′ in V_1. Normal heart

ECG 10.4 Electrocardiogram obtained from a 49-year-old woman. Incomplete right bundle-branch block with r < r′ in V_1 and T negativity in V_2 up to V_5! Atrial septal defect with left to right shunt > 60%

Complete Left Bundle-Branch Block

In complete LBBB, the QRS measures $\geq 0.14\,s$ in most cases, even without LV hypertrophy. In contrast to RBBB, in LBBB, the QRS complex is extremely deformed, because the great septal and LV vectors are directed from *right to left* and slightly upward and backward (Figure 10.3), producing a unique and somewhat bizarre QRS complex. The QRS pattern in the horizontal leads is strikingly uniform, with a broad rS complex in V_1 to V_4 (in < 20% with a QS complex) and an abrupt change to a positive deflection in V_5 and V_6 with a broad, notched (or not notched) or bifid R wave, without a q wave (ECG 10.5). Occasionally, this abrupt change can be observed between lead V_3 and V_4, or between V_5 and V_6.

In the frontal leads, the QRS axis often points to the left and upward (left axis deviation). There is a broad R wave, without a q wave, in I and aVL, and in the inferior leads III and aVF generally an rS complex and rarely a QS complex (as occasionally in V_1 to V_4), which can be confounded with a pattern of inferior infarction. However, in LBBB, the QRS is broad and the T wave is discordant positive and asymmetric in these leads (ECG 10.6), and not concordant negative and symmetric as is often seen in a previous inferior infarction.

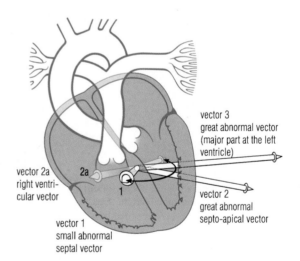

Figure 10.3 Scheme of the ventricular vectors in left bundle-branch block

vector 2a
right ventri-
cular vector

2a

1

vector 1
small abnormal
septal vector

vector 3
great abnormal vector
(major part at the left
ventricle)

vector 2
great abnormal
septo-apical vector

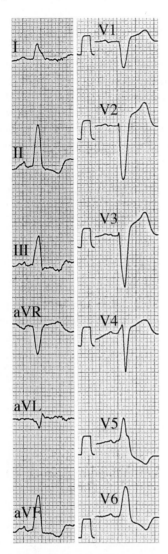

ECG 10.5 Electrocardiogram obtained from a 49-year-old woman. Left bundle-branch block, QRS duration 0.14 s (half calibration in precordial leads). Sudden change of QRS polarity from V_4 to V_5. Hypertension, left ventricular hypertrophy, pulmonary emphysema. Normal coronary arteries

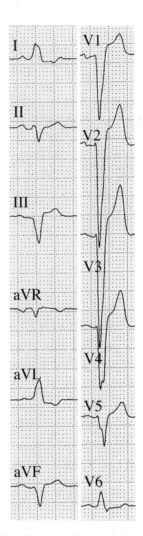

ECG 10.6 Electrocardiogram obtained from a 54-year-old man. Left bundle-branch block, QRS 0.14 s. Change of QRS polarity between V_5 and V_6, with Rs in V_6. QS in III. Dilating cardiomyopathy of the left ventricle. No significant coronary artery stenosis

Incomplete Left Bundle-Branch Block

The pattern of iLBBB is relatively rare. Its definition is a QRS duration of approximately 0.12 s and the typical behavior of the LBBB pattern in V_1 to V_6, with a sudden change from a negative QRS deflection in V_4 to a positive one in V_5 (ECG 10.7). Most of the so-called iLBBBs, without an abrupt change of QRS polarity between V_4 and V_5, are simple patterns of LV hypertrophy with prolonged QRS. In doubtful cases, for example, in the presence of a small heart, an iLBBB should be classified as complete LBBB.

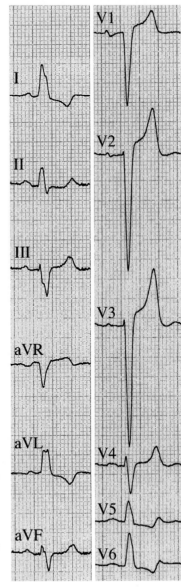

ECG 10.7 Electrocardiogram obtained from a 72-year-old woman. Incomplete left bundle-branch block (QRS 126 ms!). Change of QRS polarity between lead V_4 and lead V_5. Hypertension, left ventricular hypertrophy

Final Comments

The heart has its own and special system for conduction of electric impulses. If the function of this system is disturbed, nature looks "automatically" for another way to succeed. In the case of LBBB, the LV is activated from the RV, over the septum, bypassing the normal conduction system, in this case, the left bundle branch. If this would not happen, the LV would stand still and death would occur. Correspondingly, in RBBB, the RV would stand still without activation over the septum. Thus, the electric conduction in bundle-branch block is an example of the wonderful reserve mechanisms of nature.

Chapter 11
Bilateral Bifascicular Blocks
(Bilateral Bundle-Branch Blocks)

Bilateral bifascicular blocks, also called bilateral bundle-branch blocks, include complete right bundle-branch block (RBBB) combined with either a left anterior fascicular block (LAFB) or left posterior fascicular block (LPFB).

The prevalence of the combination RBBB + LAFB in hospital patients is 0.5%–1%, but the combination of RBBB + LPFB is at least 20 times rarer. The etiologies of these conduction block patterns are the same as in isolated fascicular blocks: coronary heart disease and cardiomyopathies of other origin, Lenègre's disease, hypertensive heart disease, heart valve operations, and rare conditions. Bilateral bifascicular blocks are clinically important because they represent potential precursors of complete infrahisarian atrioventricular (AV) block.

Right Bundle-Branch Block + Left Anterior Fascicular Block

This type of bilateral bifascicular block occurs relatively frequently (Figure 11.1). The delayed excitation of the right ventricle (by RBBB) and of high lateral portions of the left ventricle (by LAFB) alter the QRS vector loop in the frontal and horizontal plane. The electrocardiogram (ECG) is characterized by:

1. QRS duration >0.12 s.

2. Typical RBBB pattern in lead V_1 with an rsR′ complex (sometimes with a pure broad and slurred R wave, or a qR complex). The S wave in V_6 is broad (mirror image of lead V_1).

3. Frontal left axis deviation of the first 0.06 s of the QRS. Often small Q waves in aVL and I; rS complex in III/aVF/II with positive T waves.

4. Clockwise rotation of left ventricular QRS vector in the precordial leads, mostly with an rS complex and, in most cases, without a Q wave in leads V_5/V_6.

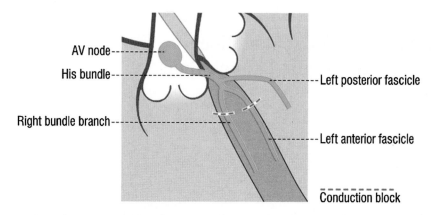

Figure 11.1 Bilateral block of the type right bundle-branch block + left anterior fascicular block. AV, atrioventricular

A slurred R downstroke in leads I and aVL, caused by a visible delayed intrinsicoid deflection, is not compulsory. Therefore, the ECG pattern in the limb leads may differ considerably, either with or without S waves in leads aVL and I. On the contrary, the QRS configuration in the horizontal plane is quite uniform (ECGs 11.1–11.3). Note that the great left ventricular vectors in ECG 11.2 are caused by left ventricular hypertrophy.

In general, the S wave in leads I and especially aVL are smaller than the S wave in lead V_6 (ECGs 11.1 and 11.2). Often, the S waves in I and especially aVL are lacking, thus imitating a left bundle-branch block pattern in the limb leads (ECG 11.3). In many cases, there is no distinct slurred R downstroke in I and aVL and occasionally the S waves are only moderately or minimally diminished in these leads. Therefore, it may be impossible in some cases to distinguish the pattern of RBBB + LAFB from that of isolated RBBB with left axis deviation. In ECG 11.4, with obvious frontal left axis deviation, an additional LAFB cannot be reliably confirmed or excluded. On one hand, the broad S waves in aVL and I and the rSR′ type in III (and aVF), with negative T waves, favor isolated RBBB. On the other hand, the *absence* of a Q wave in V_5/V_6 is quite rare in isolated RBBB and very frequent in RBBB + LAFB. ECG 11.5 shows RBBB with minor frontal QRS left axis deviation, probably *without* associated LAFB.

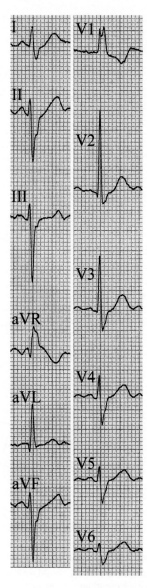

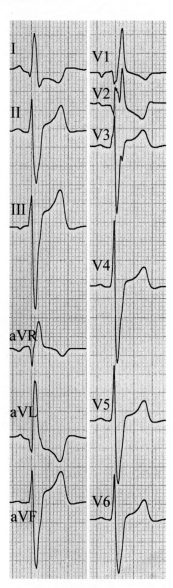

ECG 11.1 Electrocardiogram (ECG) obtained from a 73-year-old woman with hypertension. ECG: bilateral bundle-branch block. Right bundle-branch block with single and notched R in V_1. Left anterior fascicular block (LAFB): QRS left axis deviation in limb leads. Relative broad S in I but very small s in aVL. Atypical qR in V_2 (caused by a "variant" of LAFB). Typical rS complexes in V_5/V_6

ECG 11.2 Electrocardiogram (ECG) obtained from a 40-year-old woman with aortic valve replacement for severe aortic valve incompetence. Surgically induced bilateral block. ECG: bilateral block. Right bundle-branch block with rsR′ in V_1. Left anterior fascicular block: QRS left axis deviation in limb leads. Relative small s wave in I, absent s wave in aVL. rS complex in V_5/V_6, without a q wave. The great left ventricular vectors are the result of left ventricular hypertrophy. Echo: left ventricular mass 260 g/m^2

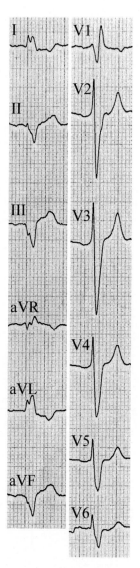 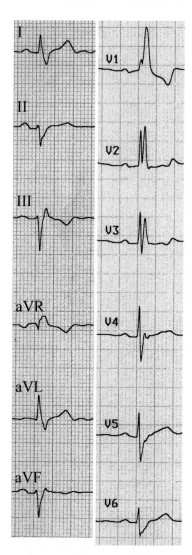

ECG 11.3 Electrocardiogram (ECG) obtained from a 68-year-old man with previous inferior myocardial infarction (MI). ECG: bilateral block. Right bundle-branch block with rsR′ in V$_1$. Left anterior fascicular block: frontal QRS left axis deviation. QS in III/aVF, the result of previous MI. Minimal s wave in I, absent s wave in aVL, with broad notched QRS. The ECG pattern in the limb leads imitates left bundle-branch block. Clockwise rotation of left ventricular vector in precordial leads. Absent Q wave in V$_6$

ECG 11.4 Electrocardiogram (ECG) obtained from a 67-year-old man with no history for coronary heart disease. Echo within normal limits. ECG: right bundle-branch block with or without associated left anterior fascicular block

ECG 11.5 Electrocardiogram (ECG) obtained from a 64-year-old man with no history for coronary heart disease. ECG: probably isolated right bundle-branch block, with rsR′ in V_1. Borderline QRS frontal left axis deviation (first 0.07 s approximately −30°). Broad S waves n I and aVL. Rs complex in V_5/V_6

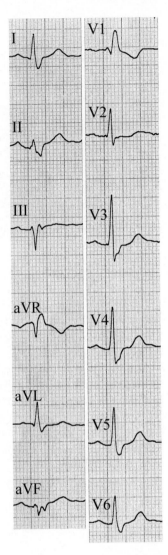

Right Bundle-Branch Block + Left Posterior Fascicular Block

This type of bilateral bifascicular block is rare (Figure 11.2). The typical RBBB pattern in lead V_1 is combined with a vertical axis of the first 0.06 s of the QRS complex in the frontal plane. The delayed activation of the inferior left ventricle portions generally leads to a visible delayed intrinsicoid deflection, a slurred R

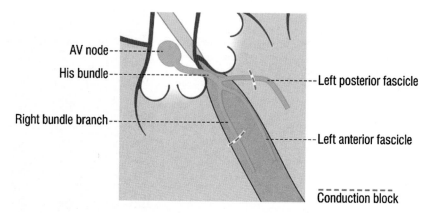

Figure 11.2 Bilateral block of the type right bundle-branch block + left posterior fascicular block. AV, atrioventricular

downstroke in leads aVF and III, and especially in lead V_6 (V_5). In these leads, the S wave is smaller and the R wave broader than usual, and the Q wave is preserved (ECG 11.6).

Without this criterion (the reduction of S and the broadening of R in leads V_6/V_5), the diagnosis of RBBB + LPFB should not be made in clinical conditions that may also lead to a vertical frontal axis of the left ventricular vector: age <40 years, right ventricular hypertrophy, lung diseases such as pulmonary emphysema, asthenic habitus, and, of course, extensive lateral infarction. Similar to isolated LPFB, RBBB + LPFB generally masks a previous myocardial infarction, reducing the Q wave in the inferior leads.

ECG 11.6 Electrocardiogram (ECG) obtained from a 72-year-old man with a surgical complication. No pulmonary disease. No history of coronary heart disease or hypertension (Lenègre's disease?). No syncope hitherto. Echo: normal left ventricular function. ECG: right bundle-branch block (RBBB) + left posterior fascicular block (LPFB) + atrioventricular (AV) block 1° (= incomplete trifascicular block). RBBB with notched R wave in V_1. Frontal vertical axis of the first 60 ms of QRS. Slurred R downstroke with consequent smaller s wave in lead V_6. The notching/slurring in leads III/aVF are probably attributable to RBBB and not to LPFB. Follow-up: in an ambulatory ECG, two episodes of AV block 2:1. The patient received a pacemaker and developed complete AV block 4 months later

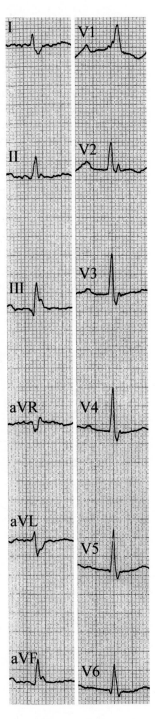

Prognosis of Bilateral Bifascicular Blocks

Bilateral bifascicular blocks represent potential precursors of a complete atrioventricular block (AV block 3°). On one hand, progression of the frequent RBBB + LAFB to AV block 3° is fairly slow (2%–4% per year), because the left posterior fascicle is generally the most resistant fascicle to any underlying disease. Thus, a pacemaker is not necessary in most cases. In patients with unclear symptoms, the duration of the VH interval may be measured, especially in cases with associated AV block 1°. On the other hand, the rare RBBB + LPFB much more often represents an immediate precursor of AV block 3°. However, the indication for pacemaker implantation depends additionally on clinical findings and symptoms such as dizziness, presyncopes, or syncopes. A Holter ECG may help to discover asymptomatic episodes of AV block 2° or 3°.

The extremely rare incomplete trifascicular block RSB + LAFB + LPFB, where an additional *medial fascicle* guarantees AV conduction, is difficult to diagnose (Figure 11.3). ECG 11.7 shows the addition of the three criteria. It represents a dangerous situation because complete AV block may develop at any time.

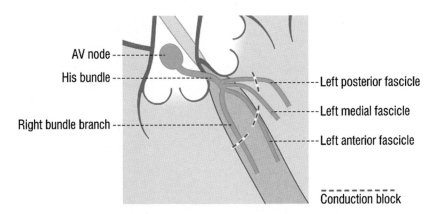

Figure 11.3 Bilateral block of the type right bundle-branch block + left anterior fascicular block + left posterior fascicular block without complete atrioventricular (AV) block. An additional medial (septal) fascicle allows or guarantees AV conduction

ECG 11.7 Electrocardiogram (ECG) obtained from a 73-year-old man. ECG (50 mm/s!): right bundle-branch block (RBBB) + left anterior fascicular block + left posterior fascicular block, without complete atrioventricular block. RBBB with rSr′ in V_1 (rsR′ in another ECG of the same patient, not shown here). Frontal axis of the first 0.06 s of QRS approximately −30°. Slurred R downstroke in leads I/aVL *and* V_5/V_6, with consecutive reduction of s wave duration. The PQ interval is not prolonged

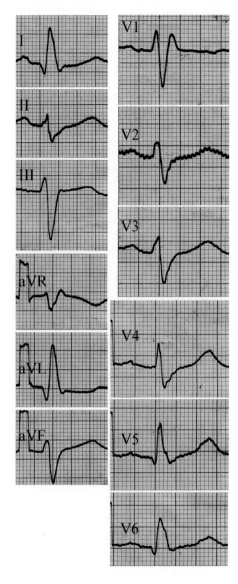

Chapter 12
Atrioventricular Block and Atrioventricular Dissociation

The atrioventricular (AV) block is linked to some important electropathophysiologic mechanisms, such as conduction slowing and escape rhythm. It is also linked to typical electrocardiogram (ECG) patterns, for example, the Wenckebach period or Mobitz block, and to other potential precursors of complete AV block, such as fascicular blocks and their combinations. Overall, the AV block, with its various degrees, is of great clinical importance.

Principally, a *conduction block* represents a prolongation of conduction time and not necessarily an absolute and fixed conduction block. Therefore, any conduction block (bundle-branch block, fascicular block, sinuatrial block, AV block) can be a variable condition that is reversible under some circumstances. AV dissociation represents a complex term and its significance depends on several conditions.

Anatomic Localization of the Atrioventricular Block

Anatomically, the AV block is localized either 1. within the AV node or in the upper part of the His bundle, in which case the expression supra-His block is used, or 2. within the infrahisarian fascicles of the right and left ventricle [right bundle branch, left anterior and posterior (and medial) fascicle] or within the lower part of the His bundle, where the His bundle spreads into the fascicles (Figure 12.1). In this case, the expression infra-His block is used.

M. Gertsch, *The ECG Manual: An Evidence-Based Approach,*
© Springer-Verlag London Limited 2009

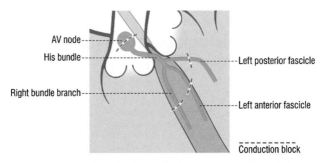

AV node----
His bundle----
                                                         ----Left posterior fascicle

Right bundle branch----
                                                         ----Left anterior fascicle

                                                         ----
                                                         Conduction block

Figure 12.1 Anatomic localization of atrioventricular (AV) block. Supra-His versus infra-His

Degrees of Atrioventricular Block

AV block is divided into three degrees: 1. In AV block 1°, every atrial impulse is conducted to the ventricles, with a prolonged PQ interval. 2. In AV block 2° (subdivided into three types), there is a change of conduction and complete AV block of the atrial impulses. 3. In AV block 3° (complete AV block), all atrial impulses are AV blocked. The actions of the atria and the ventricles occur absolutely independent from each other. If no AV nodal or ventricular escape rhythm arises, ventricular asystole occurs.

Atrioventricular Block 1°

AV block 1° is defined as PQ interval >0.20 s (ECG 12.1). Isolated AV block 1° does not represent a block, but a prolonged AV conduction, and is typically harmless and shows little or no progression during years or decades. It is also found in healthy individuals or may result from digitalis and other drugs. The prolongation of the AV conduction generally occurs in the AV node (supra-His).

Atrioventricular Block 2°

Atrioventricular Block 2°, Type Wenckebach

This type of block is relatively frequent and is characterized by an increasing PQ interval, up to one completely AV blocked atrial impulse, resulting in a short ventricular pause (ECG 12.2). This behavior is often repetitive.

The so-called Wenckebach period generally includes 3 to 4 atrial impulses (p waves). Equal to AV block 1°, AV block 2° type Wenckebach occurs in 98% within the AV node (supra-His) (Figure 12.1) and is harmless in most cases. It may progress to complete AV block in inferior acute myocardial infarction and digitalis excess.

ECG 12.1 Atrioventricular block 1°.
PQ interval 0.28 s (rate 94 beats/min)

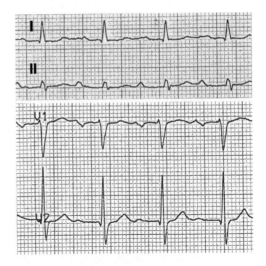

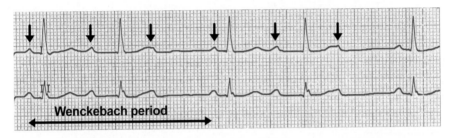

ECG 12.2 Atrioventricular block 2°, type Wenckebach. The second p of the period is partially hidden within the T wave

Atrioventricular Block 2°, Type Mobitz

This rare type of block is characterized by intermittent and sudden complete AV block of one or more atrial impulses, often without an escape beat or escape rhythm for one or more cycles. There is no increase (of the often normal) PQ interval before the ventricular pause. In the conducted beats, a bundle-branch block or a bilateral bundle-branch block is present in most cases (ECG 12.3). AV block 2° of the Mobitz type represents an immediate precursor of chronic complete AV block and is therefore dangerous. ECG 12.4 and 12.5 illustrate that in Mobitz block an escape rhythm can fail for some seconds or longer.

The block occurs distal to the His bundle in most cases (infra-His) (Figure 12.1). Patients with Mobitz block (and preexisting bundle-branch block) often have had syncope or soon will. Thus, a true Mobitz block is a clear indication for

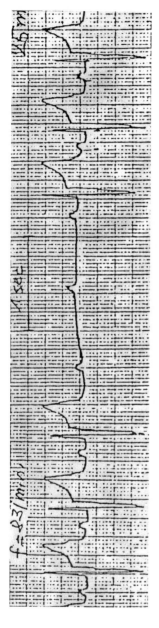

ECG 12.3 Sinus rhythm, 95 beats/min. Atrioventricular (AV) block 1° (PQ 0.2 s) and right bundle-branch block. The eighth p wave, without preceding increase of PQ interval, is completely AV blocked: AV block 2°, Mobitz type. Probably the ninth p is also AV blocked and the following QRS (see arrow) represents a ventricular escape beat (PQ before this beat: 260 ms)

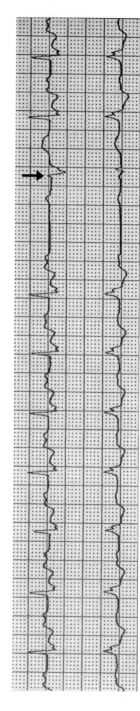

ECG 12.4 Sinus rhythm, 83 beats/min, PQ 0.21 s. Right bundle-branch block. The fourth and fifth p waves are atrioventricular (AV) blocked. There is no increase of the PQ interval before the pause: AV block 2° Mobitz

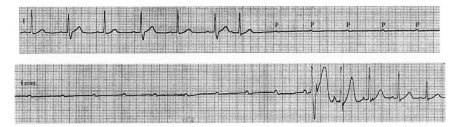

ECG 12.5   Continuous monitor strip, showing Mobitz block. Sinus rhythm, rate 62 beats/min. PQ 0.2 s. Alternating right bundle-branch block. After an atrial premature beat, 15 consecutive p waves are atrioventricular blocked, resulting in ventricular asystole of 13 s. After one ventricular escape beat, sinus rhythm continues. Note: The rate of the nonconducted p waves gradually increases, because of sympathetic stimulation. The two first T waves after the pause are artificially altered

a pacemaker. Pseudo-Mobitz occurs often in the intensive care station, especially postoperatively, is always connected with vagal stimulation and a decrease of heart rate, and the block is supra-His. Occasionally, an atypical Wenckebach block, without increasing PQ interval, is confounded with Mobitz block.

Atrioventricular Block 2°, Advanced Type

This type is also called *high degree* type. Both terms are somewhat misleading, because this type of AV block 2° is generally far from a complete AV block, in contrast to the Mobitz type. Similar to the Wenckebach type, there is a periodical change between conducted and completely AV blocked atrial impulses. The block occurs in a 2:1 or 3:1 AV block manner (up to about 8:1, especially in atrial flutter), with usually a constant and normal PQ interval (ECG 12.6). The 2:1 block means that every second atrial impulse is completely AV blocked; 3:1 means that every third impulse is completely AV blocked, and so on.

In general, AV block 2° of the advanced type is localized supra-His, and the conducted beats do not show a bundle-branch block. Progression to complete AV block is uncommon in cases without bundle-branch block with the exceptions of inferior acute myocardial infarction, digitalis excess, and rare conditions. The significance of the block type usually depends on the rate of atrial rhythm and the number of AV blocked beats. A sinus rhythm at a rate of 90 beats/min and a 3:1 AV block result in a ventricular bradycardia of 30 beats/min and impaired hemodynamics. In cases with bundle-branch block (ECG 12.7), the progression to complete AV block is more frequent. In atrial flutter, the usually present 2:1 AV block is beneficial, inhibiting an excessive ventricular rate; 2:1 AV block can also be interpreted as the shortest possible Wenckebach period. In some cases of atrial flutter, the interval between the flutter waves and the QRS complex may be irregular, because of superimposed Wenckebach phenomenon.

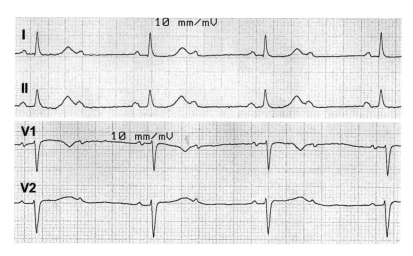

ECG 12.6 Sinus rhythm, 92 beats/min, with 2:1 atrioventricular block and ventricular rate of 46 beats/min. The conducted beats are narrow (normal QRS)

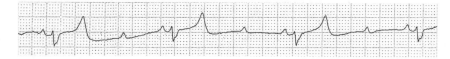

ECG 12.7 Sinus rhythm, 108 beats/min. PQ normal in conducted beats. Right bundle-branch block. Atrioventricular (AV) block 2° 3:1, ventricular rate 36 beats/min. One p wave is hidden within the apex of the T wave. The electrocardiogram changed between 2:1, 3:1, and complete AV block within minutes (not shown)

Atrioventricular Block 3°, Complete Atrioventricular Block

In AV block 3°, the conduction between atria and ventricles is completely blocked. The atria follow an atrial rhythm (mostly SR) and the ventricles, completely independently, follow an AV nodal or ventricular escape rhythm. If the escape rhythm does not arise, ventricular asystole occurs. The symptoms depend on the duration of asystole. An asystole lasting 3–6 s leads to dizziness and presyncope; an asystole >6 s leads to syncope. In patients with preexisting impairment of cerebral circulation, an asystole of 3–4 s may provoke a syncope.

A syncope caused by cardiac arrhythmias is called a Morgagni-Adams-Stokes attack (MAS attack). If asystole lasts more than 4–7 minutes, irreversible organic (especially cerebral) damage results. Longer ventricular asystole leads to death, sometimes provoked by secondary ventricular fibrillation.

Types of Complete Atrioventricular Block

As mentioned previously, there are two types of complete AV block, which differ in evolution, etiology, and clinical significance.

Infra-His Complete Atrioventricular Block

This AV block is localized distally to the His bundle (infra-His), within the ventricular fascicles and bundles, respectively (Figure 12.1). Thus, fascicular blocks, bundle-branch blocks, and bilateral bundle-branch blocks represent precursors of infra-His complete AV block (Figure 12.2). The transition from AV block 2° to complete AV block often occurs as the Mobitz type.

The rate of the ventricular escape rhythm is low, between 10 and 45 beats/min, generally 40 beats/min (ECG 12.8), and is not increased during exercise.

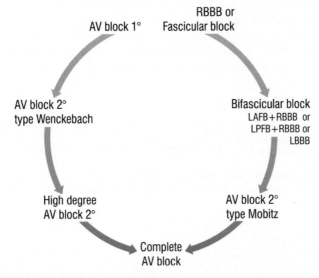

Figure 12.2 Common development to complete supra-His atrioventricular (AV) block (left) and to complete infra-His AV block (right). RBBB, right bundle-branch block; LAFB, left anterior fascicular block; LPFB, left posterior fascicular block; LBBB, left bundle-branch block

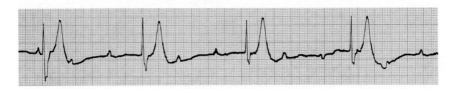

ECG 12.8 Sinus rhythm (of the atria), 75 beats/min. Complete atrioventricular block with wide QRS, rate of the ventricular escape rhythm 25 beats/min

Thus, hemodynamics are moderately to severely impaired. Moreover, the ventricular escape rhythm is not reliable in many cases and episodes of asystole are frequent.

The etiology is predominantly coronary artery disease and idiopathic fibrosis of the infra-His conduction system (Morbus Lenègre). Infra-His complete AV block is more frequent than supra-His complete AV block and is generally irreversible.

Supra-His Complete Atrioventricular Block

This AV block is localized proximally to the His bundle (supra-His), in the region of the AV node (Figure 12.1). The precursors of supra-His complete AV block are AV block 1° and two types of AV block 2°, namely, Wenckebach type and advanced type (Figure 12.2, ECG 12.9). Because the AV junctional escape rhythm is often reliable (at least during months or years) and the rate is 45–65 beats/min, episodes of asystole are rare and hemodynamics are only modestly impaired. At exercise, the rate of the escape rhythm can accelerate to 100 beats/min or more. Supra-His complete AV block is most frequently encountered in inferior acute myocardial infarction (ECG 12.10), in which the incidence is approximately 8%. In >90% of these cases, complete AV block is reversible within hours, days, or 1 week. A temporary pacemaker might be needed. Als, in digitalis intoxication, AV block is reversible

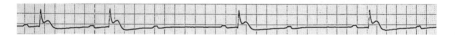

ECG 12.9 Patient with acute inferior infarction. Electrocardiogram: atrioventricular (AV) block 2° Wenckebach progressing to AV block 2° 2:1, with a ventricular rate of 23 beats/min

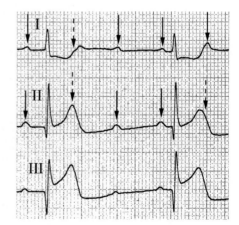

ECG 12.10 Complete atrioventricular (AV) block in acute inferior infarction (leads I, II, III). Sinus rhythm of the atria, 120 beats/min (arrows: p waves). AV junctional escape rhythm rate 44 beats/min

(after digitalis withdrawal), usually after several days. Other rare etiologies of supra-His block include congenital heart disease (with irreversible block) and infections of the heart.

Today, there is a general agreement that, principally, every patient with chronic complete AV block of infra-His localization (for short-term excess risk of syncope or sudden death) or supra-His localization (for long-term high risk) should be treated with a pacemaker. The Short Story illustrates the benign outcome of a patient with infra-His complete AV block and a very slow ventricular escape rhythm.

Short Story/Case Report

In 1980, a 72-year-old patient came on foot to our department of cardiology. The author met him occasionally at his arrival at the secretary, where he sat on a stool. He explained that he had had vertigo for several days and near syncope on the way to the hospital. The author felt his pulse on the wrist but couldn't find it. But yes, finally, there was a beat. And after 4 s, there was another beat, and after 4 s a next beat followed, and so on. The rate was approximately 15 beats/min. The ECG revealed complete AV block with a ventricular escape rhythm of 16 beats/min. The patient was informed about therapy with a pacemaker and he agreed to immediate implantation. During the intervention, he complained several times about vertigo that regularly disappeared with coughing. Each cough produced a beautiful spike of the arterial pressure (ECG 12.11, with simultaneous arterial pressure). After the implantation of a VVI pacemaker, the patient was enthusiastic about his pulse rate of 70 beats/min and insisted on going home on foot, the distance of only a 20-minute walk. His argument was that he had come on foot to the hospital with a heart rate of 16; walking home with a heart rate of 70 would be much easier. Furthermore, he wanted to surprise his wife regarding the pacemaker. A young colleague was sent to follow the patient to his home unnoticed at a good distance. During the next week, the patient came to the hospital twice for pacemaker and wound control, walking of course.

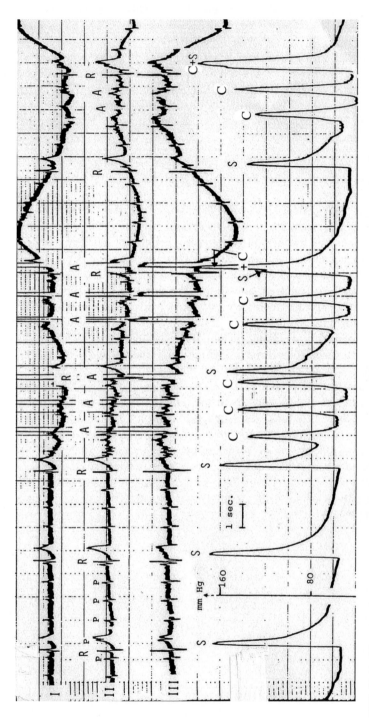

ECG 12.11 Electrocardiogram (ECG) from patient described in the Short Story. ECG leads I, II, and III written with 10 mm/s and additionally diminished. Complete atrioventricular block with an atrial rate of 66 beats/min and a ventricular rate (see R) of 16 beats/min. Lower curve: arterial pressure. Note: Coughing (C) induces impressive systolic pressure waves and artifacts in the ECG (A). S, systolic pressure induced by ventricular escape rhythm; C + S, summation of S and coughing

Atrioventricular Dissociation

The term *AV dissociation* is used on one hand as a general term and on the other hand as a special term. The general term includes complete AV block and the special types of AV dissociation (Table 12.1).

The special term is only applied to the three special forms of AV dissociation, in which the AV conduction system is not affected by a disease. Because impulse formation occurs in two centers (one in the sinus node, the other in the AV junction) nearly at the same time, each impulse only penetrates the AV conduction system. Complete conduction is inhibited by the other impulse, arriving from the opposite site. Thus, only a secondary, functional AV block is present. The ventricles follow an AV junctional center, whereas the atria are activated by the sinus node. However, in contrast to complete AV block, there is a strong time connection between the two centers.

The subdivision into three types is more or less arbitrary. All three forms of special AV dissociation are principally characterized by the same ECG pattern. The p waves are "wandering" through the QRS complexes, sometimes appearing immediately before or after the QRS, and often hidden within the QRS (ECG 12.12). The rate of the AV junction rhythm and the sinus rate only differ in small limits; over a longer episode, the rate of the two centers is the same. In contrast, in complete AV block, the p waves are "wandering" through full heart cycles, because of the higher rate of the sinus impulses compared with the rate of the independent AV junctional or ventricular escape rhythm.

Table 12.1 AV dissociation as a general term and as a special term

	AV dissociation	
Complete AV block		The three types of special AV dissociation: AV dissociation with accorochage Isorhythmic AV dissociation AV dissociation with interference

AV, atriventricular.

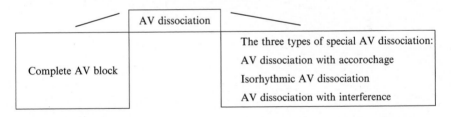

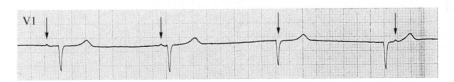

ECG 12.12 Bradycardic atrioventricular dissociation with accrochage, rate approximately 37 beats/min. The first beat is a sinus beat, the PQ time of the second p wave is shortened, the third p is hidden within the QRS complex, the last p wave appears shortly after QRS

The Three Types of Atrioventricular Dissociation

The first type is AV dissociation with accrochage, which occurs for only several beats. The second, isorhythmic AV dissociation, lasts for minutes, rarely for hours. The third, AV dissociation with interference (interference atrioventricular dissociation), is interrupted, from time to time, by conducted sinus beats, so-called *ventricular captures*.

The special forms of AV dissociation are mainly seen in healthy individuals, especially during sleep, and in athletes, and are harmless in these cases. In patients after recent heart operations or other interventions, AV dissociation may occasionally provoke a decrease of blood pressure, because of the atrial contraction against the closed tricuspid valve. The rarest type, AV dissociation with interference, is occasionally observed in organic heart disease and/or digitalis intoxication.

As already mentioned, AV dissociation is harmless in most cases, and in a post-extrasystolic beat, it is normal. Occasionally, in postoperative patients with insufficient arterial pressure, AV dissociation of longer duration may further impair hemodynamics and need intermittent atrial pacing. AV dissociation in ventricular tachycardia, present in approximately 50% of this arrhythmia, corresponds to rate-dependent functional AV block (see Chapter 26).

Chapter 13
Myocardial Infarction

Besides cardiac arrhythmias, myocardial infarction (MI) represents the most important subject in electrocardiography, because of the high prevalence and severity of the disease. Forty to fifty percent of acute and previous MIs can be recognized in the electrocardiogram (ECG) by typical ST elevation and/or pathologic Q waves, many cases with combined infarctions or with right bundle-branch block (RBBB) included. Another 20% of MIs are detectable by complex ECG patterns (with bundle-branch block or fascicular blocks) and special ECG patterns (e.g., the so-called non-Q wave infarction or new not significant Q waves).

Since the introduction of urgent percutaneous transluminal coronary angioplasty (PTCA) and fibrinolysis, accurate diagnosis of acute MI (AMI) has become more important than ever. It is therefore also necessary to recognize atypical infarction patterns and to consider the differential diagnosis of the Q wave, ST elevation, and T wave.

Etiology

More than 90% of MIs are attributable to atheromatosis of the coronary arteries with consecutive thrombosis, the latter often provoked by plaque rupture. Coronary artery spasm seems to contribute to necrosis in many cases. MI can also occur as a bystander disease in conditions such as aortic dissection, connective tissue diseases, cardiac trauma, tumors, cocaine abuse, and many others. Congenital MI, the result of coronary artery anomalies, is extremely rare.

Electropathophysiology

The description of the infarction stages in the ECG related to the electropathophysiologic evolution corresponds quite well with the real myocardial damage.

M. Gertsch, *The ECG Manual: An Evidence-Based Approach*,
© Springer-Verlag London Limited 2009

Acute Stage

Thrombotic occlusion of a coronary artery leads to ischemia, with a central zone of major ischemia, or lesion/injury. The ECG shows transmural lesion or a so-called *monophasic deformation*; the R wave, ST segment, and T wave are incorporated into a single positive deflection (Figure 13.1a).

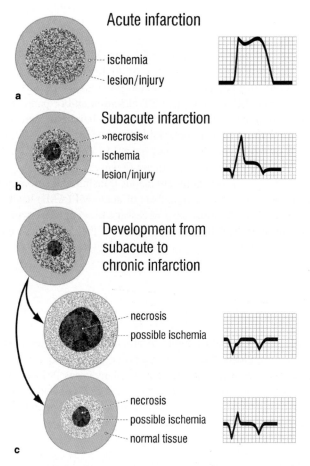

Figure 13.1   a. Acute infarction: correlation between the electrocardiogram (ECG) and the stage of myocardial ischemia. Monophasic ST deformation/"transmural" lesion = lesion/injury. **b.** Subacute infarction. Correlation between the ECG and the stage of myocardial ischemia (ST elevation = lesion, *plus* pathologic Q wave = necrosis, *plus* negative T wave = ischemia). **c.** Evolution of subacute infarction to chronic infarction

Subacute Stage

Necrosis develops in the central zone; in the ECG, a Q wave appears. The necrotic zone is surrounded by a lesion zone (minor ST elevation in the ECG), which is itself surrounded by an ischemic zone, with beginning T negativity in the ECG (Figure 13.1b).

Old Stage (Chronic Stage)

The lesion (or injury) zone is of great importance for the evolution of infarction. Figure 13.1c shows two possibilities for the evolution from subacute to previous/ chronic infarction. Either (rarely) the whole lesion zone develops to necrosis, thus increasing infarction size (Figure 13.1c, short arrow)—broad Q or QS waves are seen in the ECG; or (frequently) the lesion zone recovers partially, thus limiting the infarction size (Figure 13.1c, long arrow)—broader Q waves are seen in the ECG. In previous infarction, the ST segment has returned to the isoelectric line and the T wave is generally symmetric and negative. Often, the T wave normalizes after weeks or months.

Transmural lesion is a potentially reversible stage. Complete recovery occurs regularly in Prinzmetal's angina, attributable to reversible spasm of a coronary artery branch. In AMI, regression of lesion to ischemia or to normal myocardium is enhanced by collaterals and therapeutic procedures such as fibrinolysis or PTCA. This phenomenon is called recovering of "hibernating myocardium": a zone, formerly incapable of contraction, regains its vitality. In fact, a portion of extremely ischemic myocardium, characterized by a part of the pathologic Q wave in the ECG, may also recover. This explains why the size and duration of Q waves generally decrease during the first weeks or months after an acute infarction. A pathologic Q wave, in its strict sense, represents nondepolarizable myocardium, and not necrosis. Consequently, in rare cases, Q waves may also be completely reversible. Necrosis is never reversible, by definition.

It must be emphasized that the comments regarding the correlation between infarction size and QRS configuration are didactic. In practice, there is sometimes a good correlation; in some cases, the correlation is bad or even lacking, in "non–Q wave infarction," for example.

Why is Myocardial Infarction Not Recognizable in the Electrocardiogram in Every Case?

Approximately 70% of MIs are recognizable in the ECG, based on well-defined criteria. Approximately 30% of acute and previous MIs are not recognizable in the ECG. The reasons are: 1. small infarctions; 2. infarctions associated with left bundle-branch block (LBBB); 3. multiple infarctions, and one infarction pattern masks the other; and, last but not least, 4. electrocardiography is an indirect method.

It is therefore astonishing that so many MIs are recognized in the ECG, in many cases with reliable determination of localization and stage. Often, the clinical evolution of MI can be observed, because it corresponds (similarly to pericarditis) with an evolution of ECG alterations.

ST, Q, and T Vectors in Myocardial Infarction

Thanks to an electropathophysiologic rule, or to a gift of God, the infarction pattern at any stage appears in the directly detecting leads, independent of the preexisting QRS configuration, whether it be a qR or rS complex or another QRS complex. This fact greatly simplifies the diagnosis of "classical" acute and previous MI.

The injury (lesion) ST vector points to the region of infarction, resulting in ST elevation (Figure 13.2a). The necrosis QRS vector points to the opposite direction of the infarcted area, producing a pathologic Q wave or QS wave (Figure 13.2b). The so-called ischemia vector, in chronic ischemia, also points away from the infarction zone, resulting in negative and symmetric T waves (Figure 13.2c). For a definition of the different grades of ischemia, see Chapter 1.

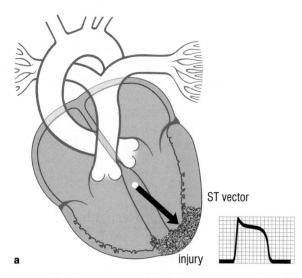

Figure 13.2 ST, QRS, and T vectors in myocardial infarction. **a.** ST injury vector. **b.** QRS vector in necrosis. **c.** T ischemia vector

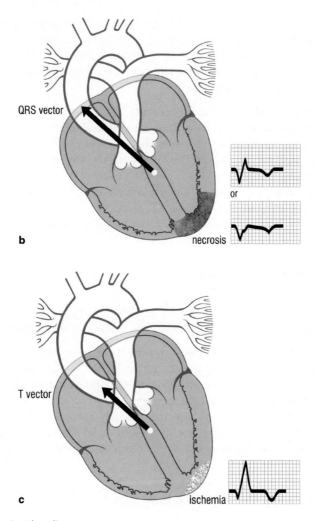

b

QRS vector

or

necrosis

T vector

c

ischemia

Figure 13.2 (continued)

Nomenclature of the Stages of Myocardial Infarction

Principally, there are four different approaches for the description of the stage of MI (acute/subacute/previous), respecting different aspects:

1. The electropathophysiologic evolution *or*
2. The international nomenclature *or*
3. The histopathologic evolution *or*
4. The clinical findings and the general clinical experience

This is a source for general confusion, because the four different approaches do not coincide with time evolution. (For details regarding the different nomenclatures for MI stages, see M. Gertsch: *The ECG*, Springer, 2004.) Below is the usual nomenclature, following the electropathophysiologic evolution, which differs from the international nomenclature:

1. Acute stage: marked ST elevation (generally >3 mm, up to 12 mm). This represents transmural lesion (also referred to as transmural injury).
2. Subacute stage: moderate ST elevation plus Q waves or QS waves. This represents minor injury and necrosis. The T wave is generally negative and symmetric, representing ischemia.
3. Chronic or old stage: "classical" Q waves (duration ≥0.04 s) or QS waves, with isoelectric ST segment. A Q wave or QS wave attributable to infarction represents necrosis. The T wave remains negative or has normalized.

International Nomenclature

1. Acute stage: ST elevation with or without pathologic Q waves
2. Subacute and old stage: pathologic Q waves, isoelectric ST segment

In other words, the ST elevation with or without pathologic Q waves corresponds to AMI, and pathologic Q waves with isoelectric ST segment (with or without negative T waves) to subacute MI and at the same time to an old MI. According to the international nomenclature, the subacute and old stage of MI cannot, therefore, be distinguished. This book uses the officially acknowledged international nomenclature. However, whenever possible, and to avoid confusion, the real age of MI, in hours, days, months, or years, is provided in the legends of the ECGs.

Localization of Q Wave Infarction

According to its localization, the infarction pattern manifests itself in different leads. If one considers the three-dimensional exploration of the cardiac vectors by the 12-standard ECG leads, it is easy to determine the localization. The direct ("optical") correlation between the localization of infarction and the exploring leads is schematically demonstrated in Figure 13.3a–f, as well as the most frequent localizations of coronary artery obstruction, for each infarction localization.

Anteroseptal Infarction

As leads V_2 and V_3 are placed over the interventricular septum, and V_4 over the apex, anteroseptal infarction will produce the typical pattern in these leads (also in V_1), according to the infarction stage (Figure 13.3a). ECGs 13.1–13.3 show an

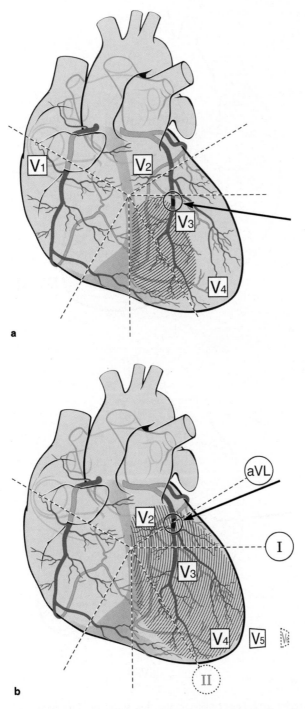

Figure 13.3 Correlation between localization of infarction and occlusion of coronary artery (arrow), and exploring electrocardiogram leads. **a.** Anteroseptal infarction. **b.** Extensive anterior infarction (anterolateral infarction)

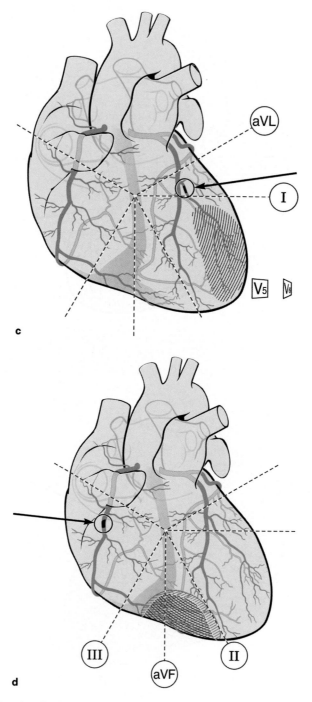

Figure 13.3 (continued) **c.** Isolated lateral infarction. **d.** Inferior infarction

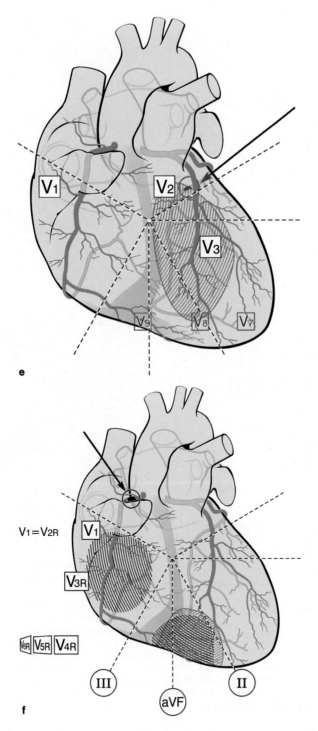

Figure 13.3 (continued) **e.** Posterior infarction. **f.** Right ventricular "infarction" (combined to inferior infarction)

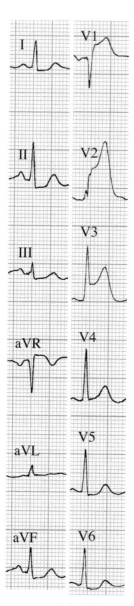

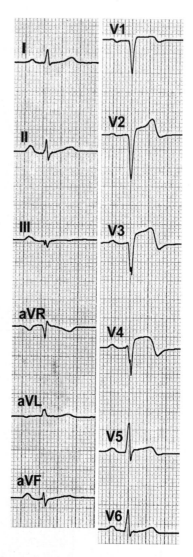

ECG 13.1 Electrocardiogram (ECG) obtained from a 51-year-old man with a 3-hour-old anteroseptal infarction. ECG: ST elevation up to 7 mm in V_1 to V_3. Coro: 90% stenosis of left anterior descending, distal to the great diagonal branch. Moderate anteroseptal hypokinesia. Ejection fraction 60%. Percutaneous transluminal coronary angioplasty with stenting. Good result

ECG 13.2 Electrocardiogram (ECG) obtained from a 42-year-old man with a 1-day-old acute anteroseptal myocardial infarction. ECG: combination of QS in V_1/V_2 and minimal R wave in V_3/V_4 (with notching) with ST elevation in (V_1) V_2 to V_5, and terminally negative T wave in V_3/V_4. Coro: 99% stenosis of left anterior descending and first diagonal branch. Apical hypokinesia, ejection fraction 70%. Percutaneous transluminal coronary angioplasty

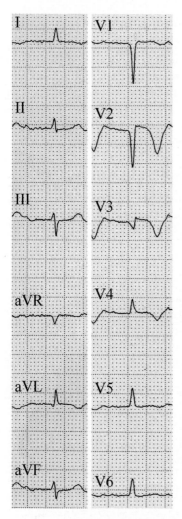

ECG 13.3 Electrocardiogram (ECG) obtained from a 94-year-old man with a 2-day-old acute anteroseptal myocardial infarction. ECG: Qr in V_2/V_3 (notching in V_4), with slight ST elevation. Negative and symmetric T waves in V_2 to V_4 and aVL. No Coro. (Note the age!)

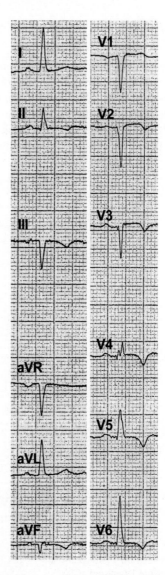

ECG 13.4 Electrocardiogram (ECG) obtained from a 63-year-old man with a 1-year-old anteroseptal myocardial infarction. ECG: QS in V_2, Qr in V_3, notched QRS in V_4 (V_3). Minimal ST elevation in anteroseptal leads. Negative symmetric T waves in V_2 to V_6 and inferior limb leads. Coro: 50% left anterior descending (LAD) stenosis (spontaneous recanalization of LAD). Anteroseptal akinesia. Left ventricular ejection fraction 60%.

AMI, ECG 13.4 an old anteroseptal infarction, involving the apex. Leads I and aVL are not influenced, because they explore antero *lateral* regions of the left ventricle (LV).

Extensive Anterior Infarction (Anterolateral Infarction)

Anterolateral infarction includes infarction of the septum, the apex, and lateral portions of the LV (Figure 13.3b). Therefore, the infarction pattern is seen additionally in the leads (V_1) V_2 to V_4, in lead V_5, and often V_6. In this infarction type, the pattern is also detected by leads I and aVL (in aVL if the high lateral portion of the LV is involved). ECGs 13.5–13.7 are examples of acute extensive anterior (anterolateral) MI, and ECG 13.8 and 13.9 are examples of old anterolateral infarction.

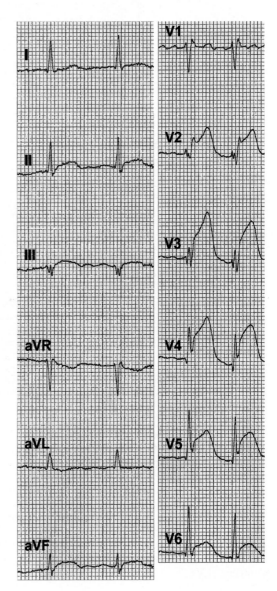

ECG 13.5 Electrocardiogram (ECG) obtained from a 64-year-old man with acute 1-hour-old acute extensive anterior myocardial infarction. ECG: atrial fibrillation (incomplete right bundle-branch block). ST elevation up to 7 mm in leads V_2 to V_6, in V_2 (V_3) arising from the S wave, and tall/broad T waves. Notched QRS in V_2/V_3. No pathologic Q waves. Coro: occlusion of left anterior descending. Anteroapical hypokinesia, ejection fraction 50%. Percutaneous transluminal coronary angioplasty

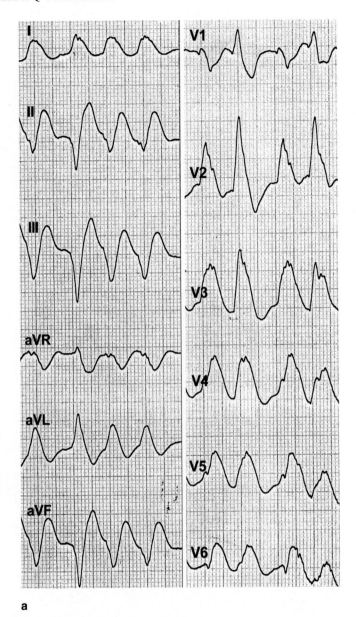

a

ECG 13.6 Electrocardiograms (ECGs) obtained from a 45-year-old man. **a.** Acute 3-hour-old acute extensive anterior myocardial infarction. Out-of-hospital reanimation (ventricular fibrillation). Potassium normal. ECG: probable atrial flutter with changing atrioventricular (AV) conduction and intermittent additional aberration. Bizarre deformation of QRS and ST ("monophasic deformation") in leads I, aVL, V_2 to V_6. QS complexes in II, aVF, and III as mirror image and not as sign of necrosis (imitation of left bundle-branch block)

ECG 13.6 (continued) **b.** ECG of the same patient 35 min later: probable atrial flutter type II with 1:2 AV conduction, ventricular rate 149 beats/min. Peripheral low voltage. QS waves in leads V_1 to V_3, pathologic Q in V_4. ST segment elevation up to 4 mm in I, II, aVL, V_2 to V_6. Coro: 20 mm long 60% proximal stenosis of the left anterior descending (LAD). Anterolateral hypokinesia, ejection fraction 58%. Interpretation: spontaneous recanalization of LAD. Percutaneous transluminal coronary angioplasty

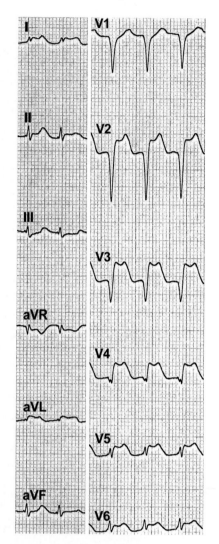

b

ECG 13.7 Electrocardiogram (ECG) obtained from a 36-year-old man with acute 3-hour-old extensive anterolateral myocardial infarction. ECG: sinus tachycardia. QS (minimal r) in V_2/V_3, relatively deep and broad Q in V_4, I, and aVL. ST elevation up to 5 mm in the corresponding leads. Coro: occlusion of the middle left anterior descending. Anterolateral hypokinesia to akinesia, ejection fraction 40%. Percutaneous transluminal coronary angioplasty

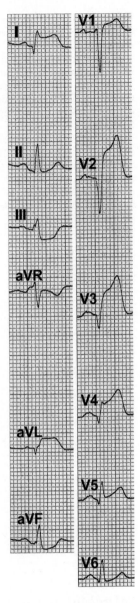

ECG 13.8 Electrocardiogram (ECG) obtained from a 66-year-old man with 4-week-old "acute" anterolateral myocardial infarction. ECG: atrial fibrillation. QS complex in leads V_2 to V_3 and pathologic Q waves in I and aVL. Reduction of R amplitude in V_4 to V_6. Slight ST elevation in leads V_2 to V_3 (V_4, I, aVL). Coro: 90% stenosis of left anterior descending (LAD) and circumflex (CX). Anterolateral akinesia, diffuse hypokinesia, ejection fraction 28%. Percutaneous transluminal coronary angioplasty of LAD and CX

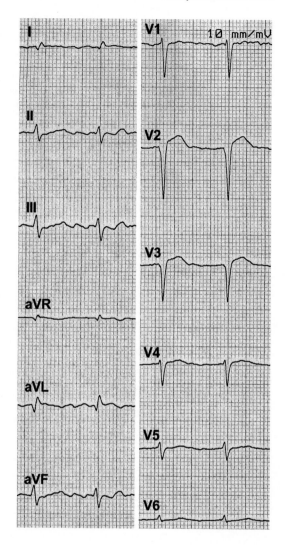

Lateral Infarction (Isolated Myocardial Infarction of the Lateral Wall)

This infarction is rare in its isolated form (Figure 13.3c). As the leads V_5 and V_6 directly explore the lateral wall, the typical pattern in these leads is seen. Depending on the infarction size, the typical signs might also be present in leads I and aVL. In high lateral infarction, the best directly—and sometimes exclusively—exploring lead is aVL. Therefore, this MI type might be overlooked.

ECG 13.9 Electrocardiogram (ECG) obtained from a 63-year-old man with 15-year-old anterolateral myocardial infarction with aneurysm. ECG: QS in leads V_2 to V_6. Peripheral low voltage. Nonsignificant Q waves in I, II, aVF, and III, rsr′ in aVL. Slight ST elevation in (V_1) V_2 to V_5. Negative T waves in inferior leads (asymmetric), and in V_6 (symmetric). Echo: extensive anterolateral aneurysm, ejection fraction 45%

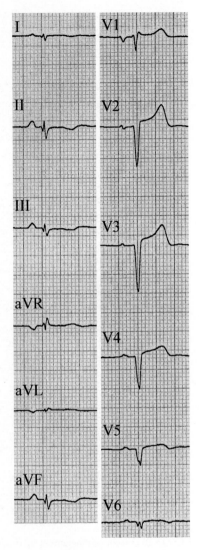

ECG 13.10 shows acute high lateral and posterior MI, with ST elevation only in lead aVL and extensive "mirror images" in other leads. ECG 13.11 shows a 4-day-old high lateral MI with a pathologic Q wave in aVL and symmetric negative T waves also in V_5/V_6 (in these leads, there are no pathologic Q waves).

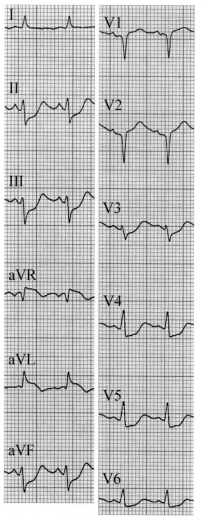

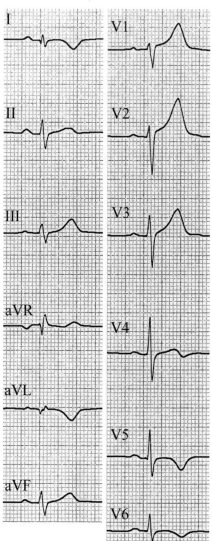

ECG 13.10 Electrocardiogram (ECG) obtained from a 78-year-old woman with acute 2-day-old high lateral/posterior myocardial infarction (MI) caused by periinterventional dissection of left circumflex (CX). Eight-month-old anteroseptal MI. ECG: sinus tachycardia. Left anterior fascicular block. ST elevation only in aVL (and aVR), with "mirror image" ST depression in II, aVF, III, and V_3 to V_6. QT interval prolonged. The old anteroseptal MI can be suspected by QS in V_1/V_2. Coro: closed left anterior descending, intermittently closed CX. Ejection fraction 60%

ECG 13.11 Electrocardiogram (ECG) obtained from a 72-year-old man with 4-day-old high lateral myocardial infarction. ECG: Qr in aVL, with symmetric T waves in aVL, I, V_5/V_6

Inferior Infarction

According to Einthoven's triangle, leads III at +120°, aVF at +90°, and II at +60° directly reflect vectors oriented inferiorly (Figure 13.3d). The pattern of inferior infarction will therefore be detected in these leads. In practice, the alterations are best seen in leads aVF and III, less distinctly in lead II. However, a q wave also in lead II favors the diagnosis of inferior infarction, whereas in pulmonary embolism, a Q wave in II is lacking.

ECG 13.12 and 13.13 show acute inferior MI. In a substantial number of cases, acute inferior MI is associated with a right ventricular (RV) infarction (see below). ECGs 13.14 and 13.15 show an old inferior MI.

Posterior ("True" Posterior) Infarction

For one particular reason, this infarction pattern is difficult to understand. According to the definition of pathologic Q waves, and referring only to the 12 standard ECG leads, the pattern is not a Q wave infarction (Figure 13.3e). We only see the mirror image of the original pattern in some of these leads. The additional posterior leads V_7, V_8, and V_9 provide the direct infarction pattern. The mirror image is seen in the opposite leads, the anterior (anteroseptal) leads V_2 and V_3, and sometimes V_1, consisting of an ST depression instead of an ST elevation and/or a great and broad R wave instead of a broad Q wave, depending on infarction stage. In absence of pathologic Q waves and/or ST elevation in the 12 standard leads, the possibility of infarction is often not considered. Thus, in the presence of the following alterations in leads V_1 to V_3, the diagnosis of posterior infarction should always be confirmed or excluded with the help of leads V_7 to V_9:

1. Single R wave and/or an Rs complex, with an R duration of ≥0.04 s
2. Isolated ST depression
3. Combination of 1 and 2

ECGs 13.16 and 13.17 show an acute posterior MI. ECG 13.18 shows an old posterior MI. An Rs complex with a relatively high and broad R wave (≥0.40 s) in leads V_1 to V_3 is occasionally seen in healthy, especially young, individuals, whereas an isolated ST depression in these leads does not exist in an otherwise normal ECG, and consequently suggests acute posterior MI. In doubtful cases and in combination with clinical signs, an echocardiogram or even a coronary angiography should be considered.

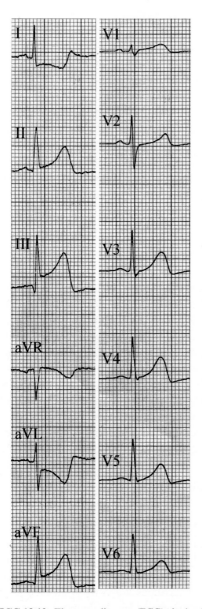

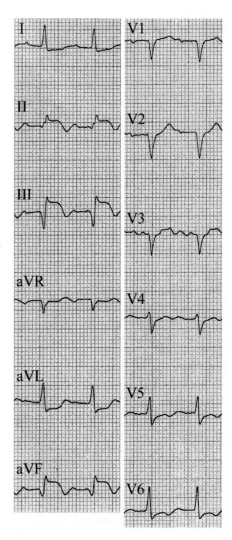

ECG 13.12 Electrocardiogram (ECG) obtained from a 63-year-old woman with acute inferior infarction, chest pain for 2 hours. ECG: ST elevation in III/aVF(II), ST depression in I/aVL as mirror image. Coro: 90% right coronary artery stenosis. Ejection fraction 62%. Percutaneous transluminal coronary angioplasty

ECG 13.13 Electrocardiogram (ECG) obtained from a 72-year-old woman with acute 24-hour-old inferior (and old anteroseptal?) myocardial infarction. ECG: atrioventricular block 1°. Pathologic Q waves, ST elevation, and T wave inversion in leads II, aVF, and III. Poor R progression in V_2 to V_4. Negative T waves in V_5 to V_6. Coro: three-vessel disease, closed right coronary artery and left anterior descending. Inferior and anterior hypokinesia, ejection fraction 45%

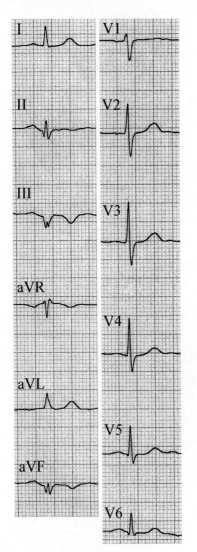

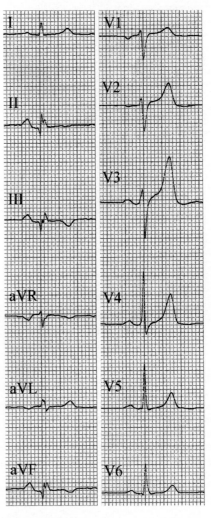

ECG 13.14 Electrocardiogram (ECG) obtained from a 67-year-old man with old inferior myocardial infarction. ECG: nonsignificant Q in II and aVF (with reduction of R wave), QS in III. Negative symmetric T waves in III and aVF. Broad R waves in V_1 to V_3 might indicate posterior involvement. Coro: three-vessel disease, inferior hypokinesia, ejection fraction normal

ECG 13.15 Electrocardiogram (ECG) obtained from a 59-year-old man with 3-year-old inferior myocardial infarction. ECG: Q in inferior leads with T inversion n III and aVF. Notched QRS in inferior and other leads. Coro: >50% stenosis of right oronary artery and left anterior descending. Ejection fraction 45%

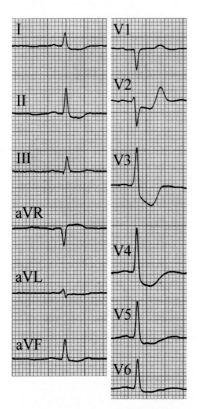

ECG 13.16 Electrocardiogram (ECG) obtained from a 60-year-old man with acute 6-hour-old posterior myocardial infarction. ECG (half calibration): enormous ST depression (mirror image of posterior ST elevation) especially in V_2 to V_6. High and broad R in V_3. Coro: three-vessel disease with occlusion of the dominating left circumflex. Ejection fraction 36%

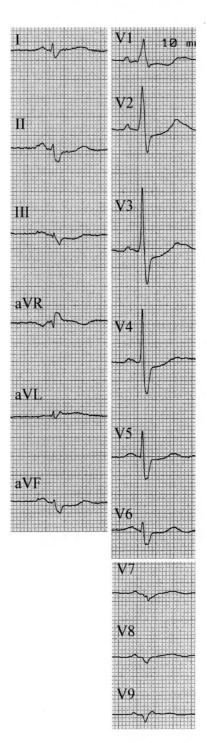

ECG 13.17 Electrocardiogram (ECG) obtained from a 74-year-old man with acute 5-day-old posterior myocardial infarction. ECG: tall and broad R wave in V_1 and V_2 (V_3), slight ST depression in V_1 to V_5, both corresponding to mirror image of alterations in the posterior leads. See: QS in V_7/V_8, Qr in V_9

ECG 13.18 Electrocardiogram (ECG) obtained from a 69-year-old man with 6-year-old posterior myocardial infarction (MI) (and 9-month-old lateral MI). ECG: tall and broad R wave in V_1 and V_2. Slightly enlarged Q waves in I and aVL, R wave reduction in leads V_5/V_6 caused by lateral MI. Coro: three-vessel disease with occluded left anterior descending (!) and 70% stenosis of left circumflex. Inferior, posterior, and lateral hypokinesia. Left ventricular ejection fraction 55%

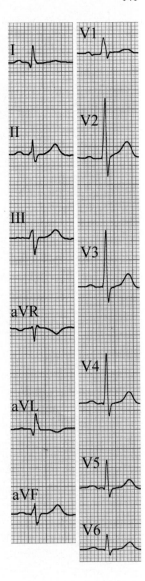

Right Ventricular Infarction

An isolated RV infarction is extremely rare (Figure 13.3f). However, an acute inferior infarction (and no other infarction type) is combined with an acute RV infarction in a strikingly high percentage, approximately 40%, generally in cases with proximal occlusion of the right coronary artery. In contrast to posterior infarction, RV infarction does not produce a mirror image in any of the standard leads. The direct infarction pattern is only detectable with the additional RV leads V_3R, V_4R, V_5R, and sometimes V_6R. Acute inferior MI combined with acute RV infarction is frequently associated with atrioventricular (AV) block of all degrees (ECG 13.19a). ECGs 13.19b, c and 13.20 show RV infarction in acute inferior MI.

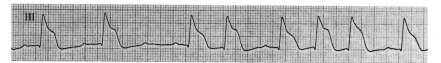

a

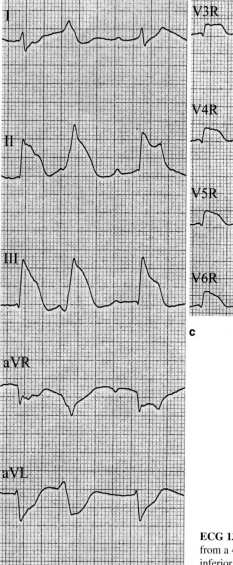

c

b

ECG 13.19 Electrocardiograms (ECGs) obtained from a 47-year-old man. **a.** Acute 12-hour-old inferior myocardial infarction with right ventricular involvement. Rhythm strip. Sinus rhythm, atrioventricular block 2° (Wenckebach and "high degree"). **b.** Limb leads: bizarre ST elevation ("monophasic deformation") in leads II, aVF, and III. **c.** Right precordial leads: small q wave and extensive ST elevation in right precordial leads V$_3$R to V$_6$R. The patient refused any intervention and died 3 days later by cardiogenic shock. Probably dominating right coronary artery

ECG 13.20 Electrocardiogram (ECG) obtained from a 63-year-old woman with acute 2-day-old inferior and anterior myocardial infarction with right ventricular "infarction." ECG: Qr in inferior leads with ST elevation and negative T waves. QS in V_1 and V_2, r reduction in V_3 and V_4, ST elevation in V_1 to V_5. QS, minimal ST elevation and T inversion in right precordial leads V_3R to V_6R

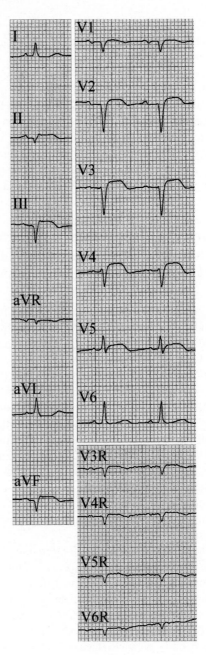

Without exception, the RV leads V_3R to V_6R *must* be applied as soon as possible in every patient with an acute inferior infarction. The medical treatment differs in the presence of RV infarction. Moreover, 48 hours after the first symptoms, the typical ECG signs for RV infarction have disappeared in 50% of the cases. One week after RV and inferior left ventricular infarction, the typical signs of RV infarction are often no longer detectable in the ECG and RV contraction has generally normalized. This proves that RV infarction is not a true infarction but represents a severe but reversible ischemia of the right ventricle, corresponding to "hibernating myocardium." However, the term RV infarction is still generally used. By far, the best, and often lifesaving, therapeutic intervention of acute inferior MI with RV infarction is immediate PTCA. The second best is thrombolysis.

Differential Diagnosis of "Classical" Infarction Patterns (Differential Diagnosis of Pathologic Q Waves, ST Elevation, and Abnormal T Waves)

The differential diagnosis of formally pathologic Q waves is extensive and includes, for example, hypertrophic obstructive cardiomyopathy, pulmonary embolism, normal variants (Q_{III}!) and, as an artifact, false poling of the limb leads (see Chapter 14).

ST elevation is seen in pericarditis (ST mostly <3 mm, without development of pathologic Q waves), as a mirror image of ST depression as a result of left ventricular overload or left bundle-branch block, in "early repolarization," in the Brugada syndrome, and other conditions. ST elevation with an amplitude of several millimeters may also be present as a normal variant in leads V_2 and V_3 (ECG 13.21). In Prinzmetal's angina, the elevated ST segment returns (with or without chest pain) to the isoelectric line, generally within a few minutes up to 20 min. Often, episodes of reversible ST elevation can only be detected in an ambulatory ECG. Of course, those patients need further evaluation with coronary angiography because significant coronary artery stenosis is common.

The so-called *non–Q wave infarction pattern* is characterized by negative and symmetric T waves (approximately 2–7 mm) in several precordial leads and in I, II, and/or aVL (ECG 13.22). The differential diagnosis of negative and symmetric T waves is extensive and includes ischemia without necrosis, subacute or chronic pericarditis, the so-called *syndrome X*, and many other conditions (Table 13.1). Tall, positive, and symmetric or symmetroid T waves are not only seen occasionally in the very early, peracute stage of MI but also in hyperkalemia and in normal patients with sinus bradycardia (in leads V_2/V_3).

In summary, for the diagnosis of MI, it is extremely important to consider the history, symptoms, and clinical findings and, in suspected acute or subacute infarction, laboratory findings such as creatine kinase (CK), CK-MB, troponin, and myoglobin. The presence of several risk factors for coronary

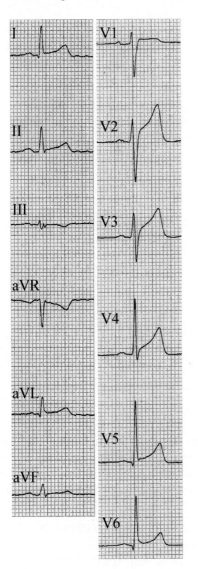

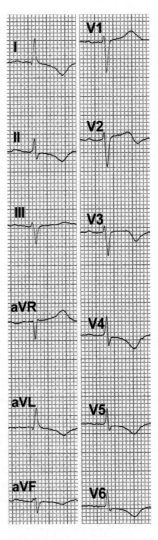

ECG 13.21 Electrocardiogram (ECG) obtained from a 56-year-old man with no heart disease. ECG: ST elevation (up to 4 mm) in leads V_1 to V_5 (V_6) and minimally in leads I, II, aVL. Normal variant

ECG 13.22 Electrocardiogram (ECG) obtained from a 72-year-old woman with 2-day-old non–Q wave myocardial infarction. ECG: sinus rhythm, atrioventricular block 1°. Symmetric negative T wave in leads I, II, aVL (aVF), and V_3 to V_6. No significant Q waves, but slightly reduced R waves in V_4 to V_6. Coro: 60% stenosis of left anterior descending (LAD), anterolateral akinesia, ejection fraction 40%. Interpretation: spontaneous recanalization of LAD. Percutaneous transluminal coronary angioplasty

Table 13.1 Differential diagnosis of acute and an old myocardial infarction in the electrocardiogram

Acute infarction	Old infarction	Classical non-Q infarction
ST ↑ without Q	Pathologic Q, isoelectric ST	T inversion only
Prinzmetal's angina	Normal variants:	Ischemia without infarction
Early repolarization	"QIII"; QS in V_2/V_3	Ventricular overload
Pericarditis	LVH "Q_{III}"	Normal variants
Mirror image of LV	False poling	Syndrome X
overload	Preexcitation (WPW syndrome)	Pericarditis (stage 3/4)
Rare conditions such as	LBBB	Myocarditis
Brugada syndrome	HOCM	Anemia
Pneumothorax	Situs inversus	Pancreatitis
	Other rare conditions*	Funnel chest
		Upright position
		Drugs
		Many other conditions†

LV, left ventricle; LVH, LV hypertrophy; WPW, Wolff-Parkinson-White; LBBB, .left bundle-branch block; HOCM, hypertrophic obstructive cardiomyopathy.
*See Chapter 14.
†See Chapter 17.

heart disease (CHD) considerably augments the probability of infarction of all stages.

Complex Infarction Patterns

The term *complex infarction patterns* means infarction in combination with the classical intraventricular conduction disturbances LBBB, RBBB, left anterior fascicular block (LAFB), left posterior fascicular block (LPFB), and bilateral blocks. A previous infarction associated with LBBB is reliably diagnosable in the presence of some high-specificity criteria such as:

1. A q wave in at least two of these leads: I, aVL, V_5, and V_6 (ECG 13.23)
2. A regression of r wave amplitude from V_1 to V_4 (ECG 13.23)
3. A notching of the S wave in V_3 to V_5 = "Cabrera sign" (ECG 13.24)

However in the absence of these signs, a previous MI cannot be excluded (low sensitivity). An AMI with LBBB may be suspected or even diagnosed by the unusual behavior of repolarization, for example, ST elevation instead of LBBB-related ST depression. In contrast, an old infarction in RBBB is generally easy to identify, in inferior and anterior localization. Identical pathologic Q waves are present as without RBBB, because necrosis influences the first 40–60 ms of the QRS complex, whereas RBBB produces alterations of the last 50–60 ms of QRS (ECGs 13.25 and 13.26). Paradoxically, an AMI in RBBB is sometimes overlooked. However, the diagnosis may be suspected, as in LBBB, on the basis of unusual ST alterations, not related to RBBB (e.g., slight ST elevation instead of ST depression in lead V_2).

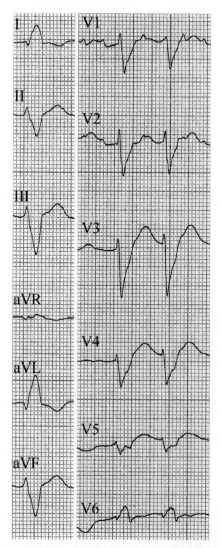

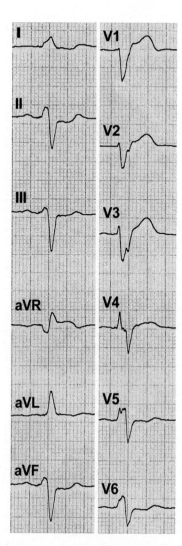

ECG 13.23 Electrocardiogram (ECG) obtained from a 70-year-old woman with 21(!)-year-old anterior myocardial infarction. Coro 5 years before: closed left anterior descending, left ventricular ejection fraction 25%. ECG: atrial flutter with irregular conduction. Left bundle-branch block (LBBB). Pathologic Q waves (in LBBB) in I/aVL, reduced R in V_5, rsR's' in V_6. Decreasing R wave from V_2 to V_5. Actual echo: ejection fraction approximately 35%

ECG 13.24 Electrocardiogram (ECG) obtained from a 75-year-old man with 18-year-old extensive anterior myocardial infarction (MI). ECG: sinus rhythm, left bundle-branch block. Pathologic notching in five precordial leads (V_2 to V_6), indicate anterior MI. Cabrera sign in V_2/V_3 (notched S upstroke). Inferior MI not diagnosable. Echo: apical dyskinesia, lateral and inferior akinesia, ejection fraction 25%

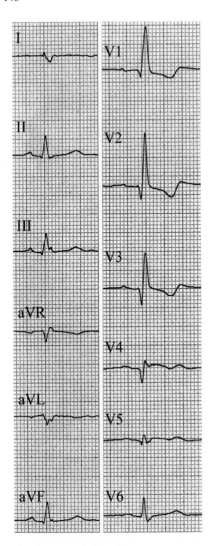

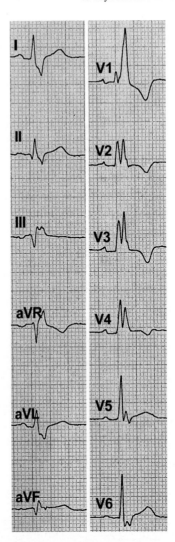

ECG 13.25 Electrocardiogram (ECG) obtained from a 70-year-old man with previous extensive anterior myocardial infarction. ECG: right bundle-branch block with pathologic Q waves in leads V₁ to V₄ (V₅) and T inversion in corresponding leads

ECG 13.26 Electrocardiogram (ECG) obtained from a 58-year-old man with bronchial carcinoma, previous inferoposterior myocardial infarction. ECG: sinus rhythm, right bundle-branch block (RBBB). Q waves inferiorly (only in III ≥40 ms), without T negativity. Tall "primary" R waves in V₂/V₃ attributed to RBBB or posterior involvement. Coro: severe three-vessel disease, closed right coronary artery, inferoposterior hypokinesia, ejection fraction 55%

LAFB may imitate or mask a previous anteroseptal infarction, or very rarely, mask inferior infarction. Extensive anterior infarction is detectable despite LAFB. LPFB represents a special condition. In practice, this overall rare conduction disturbance is almost exclusively found in inferior MI, on the one hand, whereas an inferior infarction leads to an LPFB in approximately 6%, on the other hand. LPFB often completely masks the infarction. The LPFB pattern is similar to a normal ECG; the typical alterations are subtle. ECG 13.27 shows LPFB completely masking

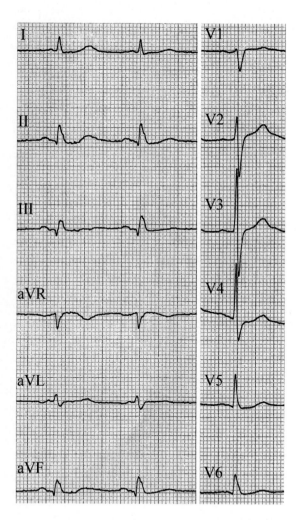

ECG 13.27 Electrocardiogram (ECG) obtained from an 81-year-old man with previous inferior myocardial infarction, masked by left posterior fascicular block. ECG: frontal QRS axis approximately +60°. Nonpathologic q waves in II, aVF, and III. Slurred R downstroke in V_5/V_6. Absent S wave in V_5/V_6. Coro: tree-vessel disease, occluded right coronary artery, ejection fraction 50%, inferolateral hypokinesia

a previous inferior MI, and ECG 13.28 provides a similar pattern in a young, healthy individual. In patients aged >40 years, with a frontal QRS axis of approximately +60°, with or without suspicious Q waves in leads III and aVF, the diagnosis should be considered, especially in patients with risk factors for CHD. (For details about LPFB, see Chapter 9.)

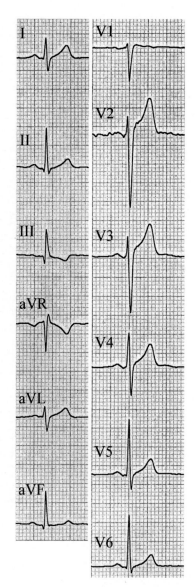

ECG 13.28 Electrocardiogram (ECG) obtained from a 27-year-old man with normal variant. No heart disease. ECG: frontal QRS axis +80°. Small Q waves in inferior leads. No slurred R downstroke in V$_6$

Special Infarction Patterns

Principally, the special MI patterns are identical to non–Q wave infarctions. Note that this definition is based on the absence of a broad Q wave, with a duration of ≥0.04 s. Therefore, MI patterns with a Q wave <0.04 s are included in the non–Q wave patterns. The special infarction patterns include the following:

1. Patterns without Q waves: a) symmetric negative T waves = classical non–Q wave infarction. b) ST depression >3 mm (ECG 13.29). Cave: in general, bad prognosis!
2. Patterns with reduction of R wave amplitude and with Q waves in the classical leads (for instance in aVF and III, in inferior infarction) with a duration <0.04 s (see Short Story).

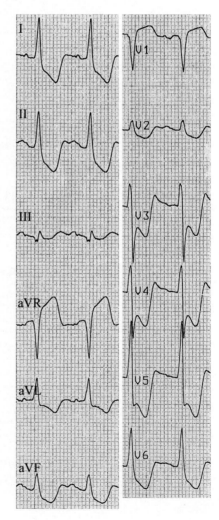

ECG 13.29 Electrocardiogram (ECG) obtained from an 82-year-old woman with angina for 2 weeks and 6-hour-old anterior myocardial infarction. ECG: excessive ST depression in leads V₃ to V₆ (7 mm in V₅) and leads I, II, aVF (aVL), with negative (or biphasic) T waves. No Q wave, except in lead III. Strange purely positive QRS configuration in V₂. Coro: 80% stem stenosis, subtotal stenoses of middle left anterior descending and circumflex, closed right coronary artery. Percutaneous transluminal coronary angioplasty/stenting of stem. Anterolateral akinesia, ejection fraction 34%. Normalization of repolarization within 1 day (not shown). Echo 3 days later: ejection fraction 50%

3. New and small Q waves (<0.04 s) in leads where they should not be present.
4. An rsR′ or rSr′ pattern in leads I and/or aVL and/or in ≥1 precordial lead V_5/V_6 (ECG 13.30). It is important to note that rsR′ or rSr′ patterns often reflect extensive anterior infarctions. Occasionally, similar patterns are found in patients with hypertrophic (nonobstructive) cardiomyopathies with indefinable intraventricular conduction disturbance.

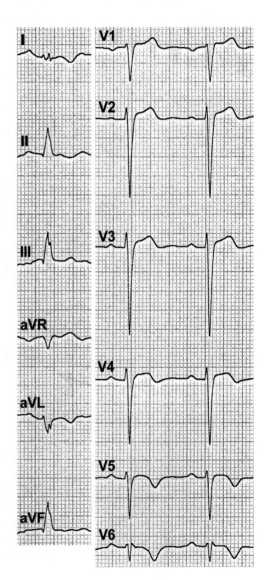

ECG 13.30 Electrocardiogram (ECG) obtained from a 57-year-old man with a 9-year-old anterolateral infarction. ECG: no pathologic Q waves, rsr′s′ in I. Notched QRS in most limb leads. R reduction from V_3 to V_6, rSr′ in V_6. Symmetric negative T waves in V_5 and V_6 (I/aVL). Vertical QRS axis attributed to loss of lateral potentials. Coro: severe three-vessel disease. Ejection fraction 24%. Anterolateral akinesia

In conditions 2–4, the presence of symmetric negative T waves in the respective leads may be helpful for diagnosis. The so-called *non–Q wave infarction pattern* represents the most important and most frequent special pattern. It is characterized (also in the acute stage!) by symmetric, negative T waves in leads V_1 to V_5 (V_6) and often I and aVL, with normal or only slightly reduced R waves (ECG 13.31). In the acute stage, ST may be minimally elevated, with above-convex configuration. The infarction may be transmural or nontransmural.

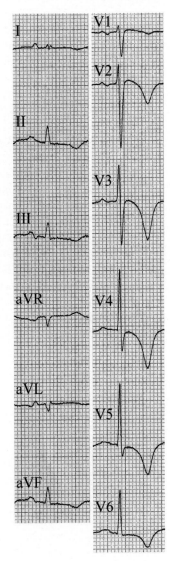

ECG 13.31 Electrocardiogram (ECG) obtained from a 69-year-old man with acute 16-hour-old non–Q wave myocardial infarction. ECG: no pathologic Q waves but deep negative T waves in all precordial and limb leads except in aVL (aVR). Coro: 90% stenosis of a dominating left anterior descending. Anterior hypokinesia to akinesia. Ejection fraction 50%. Percutaneous transluminal coronary angioplasty

In patients with non–Q wave infarction, a Q wave infarction occurs approximately 10% in the following 6 months. Therefore, an early coronary angiography is mandatory, in order to confirm the diagnosis and perform PTCA or coronary artery bypass graft, if necessary.

The Short Story describes a patient with an atypical clinical course and an ECG with new Q waves that did not fulfill the criteria of classical "infarction Q waves."

Short Story/Case Report

In March 2000, a 54-year-old colleague told the author about a slight "pulling" pain localized on the region of the left great pectoral muscle, occurring for a week during exercise with dumbbells. He also had some general malaise. He denied having risk factors for CHD. His blood pressure was 170/100 mmHg at rest, the ECG revealed a "special" infarction pattern with inferoposterior localization, without significant Q waves in the inferior leads, but with suspect symmetric negative T waves (ECG 13.32a). The family doctor instantly faxed the ECG obtained at a checkup 3 years before, which was completely normal (ECG 13.32b).

The stress test revealed an excellent work capacity (rate of 160 beats/min at 17 MET); however, the strange "muscular pain" could be reproduced. Heart enzymes were normal. Coronary angiography performed on the next day showed a complete proximal obstruction of a great circumflex artery with some collateralization, and LV angiography showed a minor circumscript hypokinesia inferoposteriorly, with a normal ejection fraction of 70%. The other coronary arteries were normal. Desobstruction and stenting were performed, with a good result. On reexercise test the next day, no pain occurred. Risk factors such as moderate hypertension, hypercholesterinemia, and moderate adipositas were treated. Surprisingly, the "special" ECG pattern unveiled the infarction better than LV angiography in this case.

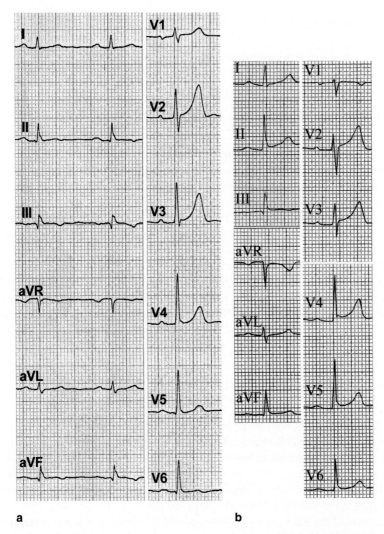

a   b

ECG 13.32 Electrocardiograms (ECGs) obtained from a 57-year-old man described in the Short Story. **a.** ECG: nonsignificant Q waves (<0.04 s) in II, aVF, III, with symmetric negative T waves. R waves in V_1 to V_3 ≥0.04 s, with high symmetric T waves. Overall, the ECG suggests previous posteroinferior infarction. **b.** Normal ECG 3 years before

Complications of Acute Myocardial Infarction

A brief overview of the complications of AMI is provided below.

Arrhythmias and Conduction Defects

Arrhythmias represent the most frequent direct complications of AMI, including ventricular premature beats, monomorphic ventricular tachycardia and ventricular fibrillation, AV blocks of all degrees, and ventricular tachycardia of the type torsades de pointes, in some cases.

In inferior infarction, especially in combination with RV infarction, complete AV block of suprahisarian localization develops in approximately 12% of the cases and generally regresses spontaneously over AV block 2° and 1°, to normal AV conduction within days. Definitive pacing is rarely required. Complete infrahisian AV block is rare, indicates severe damage of the LV, and is seen in extensive anterior infarction. The appearance of a new RBBB, LBBB, or bilateral block in the course of acute infarction is observed in 0.5%–8% of cases; RBBB occurs more frequently than LBBB. A new LAFB is astonishingly rare, at >5%.

Nonarrhythmic Complications

Ventricular aneurysm is not rare in anterior infarctions. Persisting ST elevation of >1 mm in >3 anterolateral leads, in anterior Q wave infarctions, represents a reliable sign for aneurysm. However, in many aneurysms of the anterior LV wall, ST elevation is missed. For unknown reasons (perhaps because of the absence of the "proximity effect" in the limb leads), inferior aneurysm is only exceptionally detectable by persisting ST elevation in leads aVF, III (and II).

For rupture of the left ventricular free wall and for ventricular septal perforation, there are no reliable ECG signs. In some cases, a "second" ST elevation may announce imminent wall rupture. The common nonarrhythmic complications of MI such as shock, acute mitral regurgitation caused by rupture of subvalvular tissue and ventricular septal defect, are diagnosed on the basis of typical clinical findings and with the help of echo/Doppler, the Swan-Ganz catheter (determination of right heart O_2 saturation in the case of septal perforation), or conventional heart catheterization.

Chapter 14
Differential Diagnosis of Pathologic Q Waves

For decades, the Q wave (Q > R), the QS wave (purely negative QRS complex), and the q wave (Q < R) have engrossed not only cardiologists but also many other physicians in different disciplines of medicine. A reappraisal of this important subject is appropriate.

Definition of the Normal Q Wave

The normal Q wave is always a q wave, which means that it is smaller than the following R wave (ECG 14.1). The normal q wave is attributed to the depolarization of the interventricular septum. Its duration is usually a few to 15 ms and never exceeds 20–25 ms (excluding the normal variants of "Q_{III}," QS in V_1/V_2). Often, there is no q wave in many leads because the projection of the septal vector on these leads is positive and therefore is manifested in the first 15 ms of the R wave. In the normal electrocardiogram (ECG), in lead aVR, there is always a predominantly negative QRS complex. Lead aVR is situated at −150° in the frontal plane and shows a mirror image of the usual QRS complex. We find a Qr or even a QS complex or an rS or rSr′ configuration.

Definition of the Pathologic Q Wave

The pathologic Q wave is defined as a Q wave (or first negative deflection of QRS) with a duration of ≥0.04 s. The deepness of the Q wave is not important.

Pathologic Q Waves in Myocardial Infarction

Of course, the diagnosis of myocardial infarction is often made in the presence of smaller Q waves, for instance in cases of broader Q waves than before, in cases of new Q waves, or if one or several Q waves appear in leads where they are unusual.

M. Gertsch, *The ECG Manual: An Evidence-Based Approach*,
© Springer-Verlag London Limited 2009

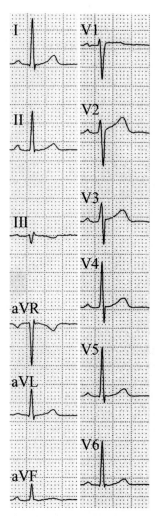

ECG 14.1 Electrocardiogram (ECG) obtained from a 35-year-old man with lung carcinoma. ECG: normal, with small q waves in leads I/aVL and V_5/V_6

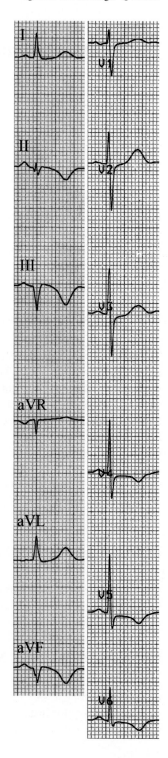

ECG 14.2 Electrocardiogram (ECG) obtained from a 69-year-old woman with a 4-day-old inferior infarction. ECG: QS in leads III/aVF, qrs in lead II, combined with deep symmetric negative T waves. Slight ST depression and negative T waves in V_4 to V_6. QT prolonged. Coro: great right coronary artery closed. Percutaneous transluminal coronary angioplasty

Also, infarctions without any Q wave are possible, in the so-called non–Q wave infarction. Typical for a myocardial infarction is its dynamic behavior. Generally, an infarction shows an evolution from the acute stage with ST elevation, which is accompanied by chest pain and elevated levels of creatine phosphokinase and troponin, over a subacute stage with the appearance of pathologic Q waves, to the old stage with persistence of Q waves, normalization of the ST segment, and often negative T waves that are generally symmetric. ECG 14.2 shows a previous inferior infarction. The Q wave in myocardial infarction is attributed to necrosis.

Pathologic Q Waves in Other Conditions

Pathologic Q waves of an etiology other than myocardial infarction are characterized by obvious Q waves of different duration and variable deepness, sometimes in leads where they should not be present. These abnormal Q waves are caused by the projection of QRS on the different leads (the "Q_{III}" as normal variant), to septal hypertrophy [as in some cases of hypertrophic obstructive cardiomyopathy (HOCM)], to abnormal heart position, such as situs inversus, or in other instances interpreted as "of unclear etiology." However, it is obvious that in those cases, such as in amyloidosis or in certain cardiomyopathies, the underlying disease has produced a "myocardial scar," or necrosis, resulting in a loss of ventricular electric forces.

Patterns with Pathologic Q Waves Not Attributable to Myocardial Infarction

Left Ventricular Hypertrophy

Left ventricular hypertrophy (LVH) produces a Q or even QS in III (avF). In rare cases of pure severe aortic valve incompetence, there is a small (25 ms) but very deep Q (up to 2.5 mV) in V5/V6.

False Lead Poling

The erroneous exchange of the upper limb leads (left versus right) is the most frequently seen by far and the easiest to recognize. The whole electric cycle in lead I shows the mirror image of the normal pattern. There is not only a "pathologic" Q, but the R wave is equally inverted and the p wave is negative (ECG 14.3). A glance to the precordial leads will rule out any anterior infarction and a situs inversus as well, which is very rare (see "Other Conditions for Pathologic Q Waves" below). For all possible false poling in vertical and left electric heart position, see the comprehensive book, M. Gertsch, *The ECG*, Springer, 2004.

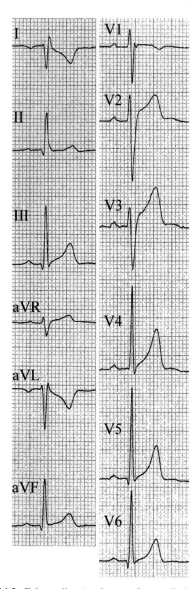

ECG 14.3 False poling (exchange of upper limb leads)

Left Bundle-Branch Block

Occasionally, in frontal QRS left axis deviation, QS in III (aVF) with positive asymmetric T waves is seen in left bundle-branch block. Rarely, QS in V_1 to V_4 (often minimal r waves) is seen. QRS duration is always broadened to ≥ 0.14 s (see Chapter 10).

Preexcitation (Wolff-Parkinson-White Syndrome)

In preexcitation over a posteroseptal pathway, the delta wave and the QRS are usually negative in III/aVF. The correct diagnosis is easy (see Chapter 24).

Hypertrophic Obstructive Cardiomyopathy

The ECG in HOCM shows a broad spectrum of patterns. Slightly pronounced q waves may be present in leads V_5/V_6 (I/aVL) (see ECG 14.4). These Q waves may reach a duration of 0.04 s or, very rarely, be giant to a degree of fully dominating the ventricular depolarization leading to negative QRS complexes in all leads except aVR (ECG 14.5).

Many HOCM ECGs, however, are not suspicious by striking Q waves but show only signs of common LVH, a left bundle-branch block, or, surprisingly enough, are completely normal, even in the presence of a substantial intraventricular systolic gradient.

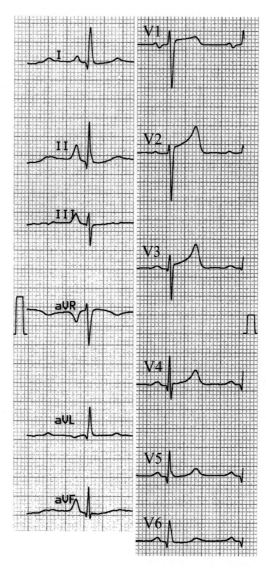

ECG 14.4 Electrocardiogram (ECG) obtained from a 40-year-old man with hypertrophic obstructive cardiomyopathy (systolic mean gradient 50 mmHg). ECG (half calibration in precordial leads!): atypical left atrial enlargement ("p pseudo-pulmonale"). Q waves pronounced in V_4 to V_6 (V_3). Sokolow index positive (44 mm), ST elevation in V_1 to V_4 (up to 4 mm)

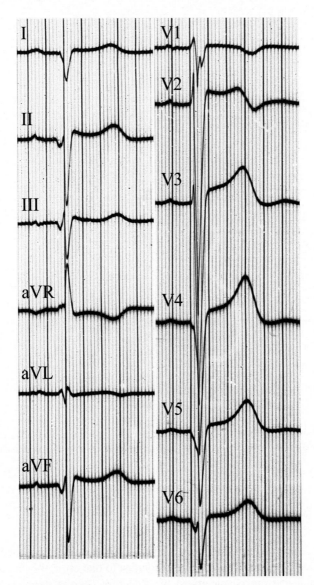

ECG 14.5 Electrocardiogram (ECG) obtained from a 22-year-old man with severe hypertrophic obstructive cardiomyopathy. ECG (50 mm/s): sinus rhythm. Striking QRS vector in the limb and precordial leads. Frontal QRS axis approximately −130°, with a positive QRS complex only in lead aVR. Giant S waves in V_2/V_3. QS complexes in leads I, II, and V_4 to V_6, as in extensive lateral myocardial infarction (positive discordant T waves, however)

Normal Variants

Because of projection, q waves or even a QS in leads III (aVL) or V_2 and V_3 are rarely found in normal subjects, even with correct lead placing (ECG 14.6).

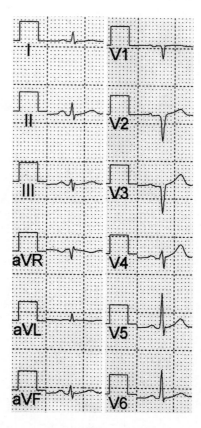

ECG 14.6 Electrocardiogram (ECG) obtained from a 74-year-old man with no heart disease, no risk factors for coronary heart disease. ECG (half calibration): QS in V_1/V_2, minimal r wave in V_3. Echo: normal

Situs Inversus

Similarly to false poling of the upper limb leads, situs inversus provokes an inversion of the electric cycle in lead I. But in contrast to that error, the precordial leads are not normal and are characterized by a decrease of the R waves and by an increase of the S waves from V_2 to V_6. Corresponding derivations at the right thoracic side reveals a normal ECG, thus assuring the correct diagnosis.

Congenital Corrected Transposition of the Great Arteries

In this rare congenital heart disease, the ventricles are reversed and the ventricular septal depolarization occurs from right to left. As one consequence, there are small q waves, generally a qrS complex in leads V_1/V_2, and no q waves in V_5/V_6, in only about 30% of the cases.

Other Conditions for Pathologic Q Waves

Pathologic Q waves have occasionally been described after pneumectomy, after pericardectomy, in pneumothorax, and in peripheric muscular dystrophy type Duchenne associated with hypertrophic cardiomyopathy, and, in the case of Morbus Steinert, a circumscript damage (scar with q waves) in the left posterolateral region. Also, in cardiac amyloidosis, pathologic Q waves have occasionally been found.

Can a Pathologic Q Wave Provide a Clue for an Atrial Alteration?

In massive acute pulmonary embolism or in severe mitral stenosis with consecutive tricuspidal incompetence, a QR or Qr complex in lead V_1 might be observed. This is not a sign for right ventricular hypertrophy but indicates severe right atrial dilatation. Thus, an alteration of the ventricular complex, a QR type, is a sign for right atrial dilatation, even in the presence of atrial fibrillation (ECG 14.7). A reasonable explanation for this unique phenomenon would be complex.

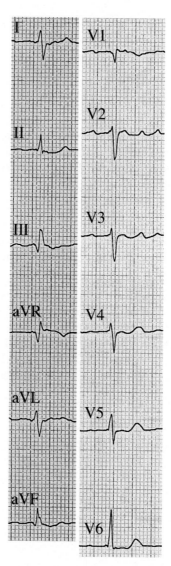

ECG 14.7 Electrocardiogram (ECG) obtained from a 72-year-old woman with severe mitral stenosis with pulmonary hypertension, right ventricular failure, and tricuspid regurgitation. Mitral valvulotomy 24 years previously. ECG: atrial fibrillation. Q wave (Qr complex) in V_1, because of right atrial enlargement. The Q wave disappeared after diuretic therapy and regression of the heart size

Chapter 15
Acute and Chronic Pericarditis

Compared with myocardial infarction, pericarditis is a relatively rare disease that is more often encountered in general practices than in hospitals. Acute pericarditis is generally of viral or unknown etiology. The main symptom is a sharp, rarely dull pain of sudden onset in the heart region, varying with breathing and in different body positions. The pain might radiate to the neck and scapular region. Electrocardiogram (ECG) alterations can be detected in up to 90% of the cases, if serial ECGs are available.

Etiology

Acute pericarditis is generally of unknown origin (in which case it is called "idiopathic pericarditis") or of viral etiology. Chronic pericarditis is associated with many conditions. A summary of etiologies for acute/subacute pericarditis is presented in Table 15.1. (For chronic pericardial disease, see Table 15.3.)

Acute Pericarditis

In pericarditis, four stages can be distinguished, theoretically. Not all stages are always present in the same patient.

1. Peracute stage: PQ depression
2. Acute stage: ST elevation (*plus* PQ depression in approximately 50%), positive T wave
3. Intermediate stage: ST and PQ isoelectric, flattened T waves
4. Subacute stage: Negative T waves, ST and PQ isoelectric
5. Postpericarditis: Normal ECG

Table 15.1 Etiology in acute pericarditis

1. Common
   - Idiopathic
   - Viral: Coxsackie A and B, echovirus, adenovirus
   - Bacterial: staphylococcus, streptococcus, pneumococcus
   - Myocardial infarction
   - Heart surgery
   - Chest trauma

2. Rare
   - Viral: mononucleosis, varicella, mumps, hepatitis B. Ebstein-Bar
   - Bacterial: meningococcus, *Neisseria* (*meningitidis, gonorrhoica*), *Klebsiella, Brucella, Escherichia coli, Salmonella, Proteus, Bacteroides fragilis, Pseudomonas, Clostridium, Fusobacterium, Bifidobacterium*, gram-negative sepsis
   - Pulmonary embolism (in 4%)
   - Fungal: candida, histoplasmosis, and others
   - Other infections: Lyme disease, toxoplasmosis, mycoplasma, echinococcus, amebiasis, leishmaniasis (kala-azar)
   - Acute rheumatic fever
   - Other conditions: dissecting aortic aneurysm. Radiation. Pacemaker implantation. Drugs: procainamide, phenytoin, hydralazine, phenylbutazone, doxorubicin, clozapine, penicillin with eosinophilia. Eosinophilic.

Peracute Pericarditis

PQ depression is a slightly descending segment between the end of the p wave and the beginning of the QRS complex. It is seen as an isolated ECG sign at the very early stage in approximately 50% at best, in our experience (ECG 15.1). This alteration is extremely rare in acute myocardial infarction (AMI). The ECG 15.2 shows the more common combination of PQ depression with ST elevation in stage 2 (acute) pericarditis.

Acute Stage

The most striking alteration is an ST elevation that generally does not exceed 2.0 mm and may be present in the majority of the 12 standard leads, with the exception of lead aVR, where ST is always depressed, and occasionally of lead V_1, where ST might be depressed. In the precordial leads, the ST elevation is accentuated more midprecordially (V_3 to V_5) or more laterally (V_5 and V_6). In contrast to the pattern in AMI, where the ST elevation generally arises from the R downstroke and is mostly of higher amplitude, the ST segment frequently arises from the S wave, in the midprecordial leads. However, in the limb leads and in the lateral leads V_5/V_6, the ST elevation might arise from the R downstroke, as in acute infarction. And in AMI, ST elevation sometimes arises from the S wave (e.g., in V_2 to V_4). In approximately 50% of the cases, PQ depression is still present in stage 2.

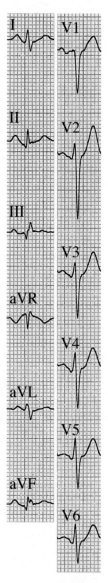

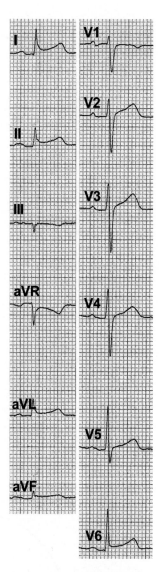

ECG 15.1 Electrocardiogram (ECG) obtained from a 53-year-old man. ECG 6 hours after onset of acute chest pain. Early acute stage of pericarditis with PQ depression in I, II, aVF, and V_1 to V_6

ECG 15.2 Electrocardiogram (ECG) obtained from a 74-year-old man who had liver treatment. Subacute pulmonary embolism with small pleural and pericardial effusion. ECG: frontal ST vector +30°, with ST elevation in aVL, I, II, and aVF. Only slight ST elevation in (V_2/V_3/V_4) V_5/V_6. Note also PQ depression in I, II, aVF, and V_3 to V_6 .

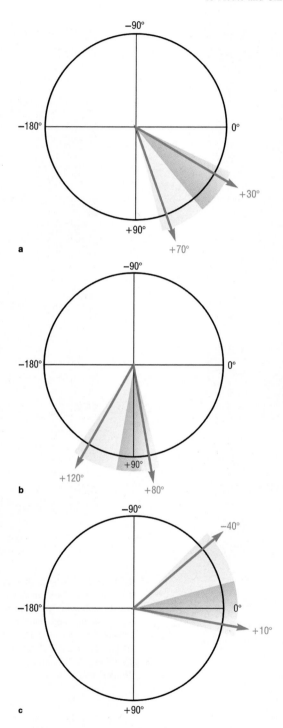

Figure 15.1 a. Frontal ST vector in acute pericarditis. **b.** Frontal ST vector in acute inferior myocardial infarction (MI) **c.** Frontal ST vector in acute anterior MI

How then, does one reliably distinguish acute pericarditis from AMI with ST elevation? A very important criterion is the frontal ST vector. In pericarditis, it is situated between +30° and +70° (Figure 15.1a). Thus, the ST segment is elevated in leads aVF, II, and I, a condition that is never seen in AMI. The ST vector is between +80° and +120° in inferior AMI (Figure 15.1b) and between +10° and −40° in extensive anterior AMI (Figure 15.1c).

Also, in contrast to the ECG pattern of myocardial infarction, the ECG during the evolution of pericarditis never shows a development of pathologic Q waves or a reduction of the R waves. Moreover, as mentioned previously, the amplitude of ST elevation in acute pericarditis is modest (2.5 mm at most), whereas it is generally >3 mm in AMI and can reach 8–10 mm. The often cited formal difference of ST elevation (concave, convex) is unreliable, especially in ST elevation of minor degree.

A special, almost specific sign of acute pericarditis is the so-called *stork leg sign* (Figure 15.2). This is a short, positive, and small deflection (0.2–1 mm) in the region of the J point, at the end of the QRS complex, and the beginning of the ST segment. The term's name derives from its unusual pattern: If the QRS complex is reversed by 180°, it is similar to a stork standing on one leg (the inverted R wave), with the other leg drawn to the body (the small "J point deflection"; see arrow in ECG 15.4). The stork leg sign is generally seen in leads V_4 to V_6, rarely inferiorly, in approximately 30%–40%. Otherwise, this sign is seen in hypothermia, and in its abortive form (amplitude about 0.1 mm) as a normal variant.

However, it is optimal to diagnose pericarditis on the basis of several criteria, and to discriminate acute pericarditis from AMI. Table 15.1 shows the etiology in acute (subacute) pericarditis, and Table 15.2 summarizes the respective differences between acute/subacute pericarditis and myocardial infarction.

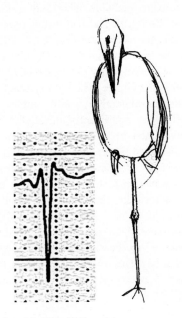

Figure 15.2 Stork leg sign (designed by Ursula Gertsch)

Table 15.2 Acute/subacute pericarditis and myocardial infarction

Acute pericarditis versus acute ST↑ myocardial infarction (AMI) in the ECG		
	Acute pericarditis	AMI
PQ depression	In about 50%	No
Voltage of ST elevation	0.5–2.0 mm	Generally >3 mm
Frontal ST vector	+30° to +70°	Anterior AMI: +10° to −40°
		Inferior AMI: + 80° to +120°
Pathologic or new Q waves	No	Yes or not yet
Stork leg sign	In 30%–40%	No
ST depression in V_1	In about 10%	Only as "mirror image" of acute posterior or inferoposterior infarction, often in V_2 (V_1/V_3)

AMI, acute myocardial infarction; ECG, electrocardiogram.

For general differential diagnosis of ST elevation, see Chapter 13. The frontal ST vector in acute pericarditis is between +30° and +70° in 80%–90%. ECG 15.3 shows an exception in a 79-year-old woman with a frontal ST vector of +10°. The Short Story illustrates a typical case of acute pericarditis in a colleague.

Short Story/Case Report

On February 17, 2000, the author received a phone call from a close friend and professor in psychosomatic medicine, who spent a skiing holiday in a little village. For several days he felt ill and had a dull retrosternal pain that at times radiated to the scapula, the neck, and both ears. The pain increased by deep breathing and under the Valsalva maneuver. Despite feeling ill, the patient performed about 20 km of cross-country skiing a day. On the author's proposition, he visited a physician in the village, who obtained an ECG. In the opinion of the colleagues, a subacute inferolateral myocardial infarction could not be excluded [creatine kinase (CPK) was significantly elevated: 648 μ/L, normal up to 195, troponin value, received later from an external laboratory, was normal]. On the basis of the ECG transmitted by fax, the author could appease both colleagues. The frontal ST vector was +70°, the stork leg sign was present, and the ST elevation arose from the s wave (ECG 15.4). The further evolution was uneventful. Two weeks later, the echocardiogram revealed a small pericardial effusion over the right ventricle, the ECG had normalized, and the patient felt well again. Serum diagnostics were not made (as usual in a physician-patient); the elevated CPK value was attributed to the skiing. Coronary angiography was not performed. Why should it be? The patient had no risk factors for coronary heart disease, except stress!

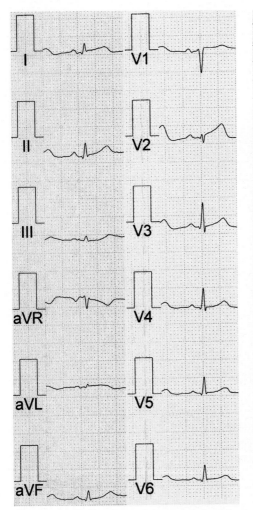

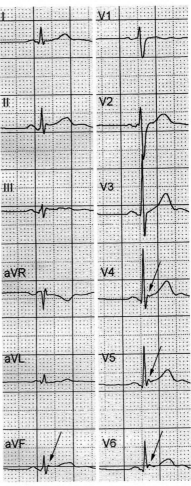

ECG 15.3 Electrocardiogram obtained from a 79-year-old woman. Viral pericarditis with an abnormal frontal ST vector of +10°

ECG 15.4 Electrocardiogram (ECG) obtained from the 62-year-old man described in the Short Story. Idiopathic acute pericarditis. ECG: frontal ST vector +50° ST elevation in I, II, aVF, III, and V_4 to V_6 (V_2/V_3). Stork leg sign in aVF and V_4 to V_6 (↓). Minimal PQ depression in V_4/V_5 and in some limb leads (short PQ interval)

Stage 3: Intermediate State of Pericarditis

In this stage, the ST elevation returns to the isoelectric line, and the T waves are flat or show beginning negativity (ECG 15.5). Without preceding ECGs, it is impossible to make a diagnosis.

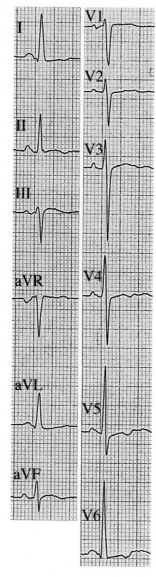

ECG 15.5 Electrocardiogram (ECG) obtained from a 60-year-old woman with subacute viral pericarditis. ECG: negative T waves in II and V_3 to V_6

Stage 4: Subacute Pericarditis

Negative T waves are typical, generally symmetric (as in ischemia), and best detectable in the precordial leads (ECG 15.6). They may last for days or several weeks. T negativity can only be interpreted correctly if previous ECGs demonstrate the typical signs of acute pericarditis.

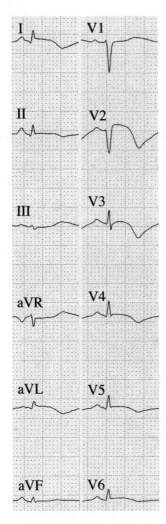

ECG 15.6 Electrocardiogram (ECG) obtained from a 79-year-old woman. Subacute viral pericarditis with symmetric T waves in I, aVL, II, V_2 to V_5 (V_6)

Arrhythmias are rarely provoked by pericarditis (except sinus tachycardia). If arrhythmias occur, one has to look for coexisting organic heart disease. This may be concomitant myocarditis (rather rare with obvious myocardial damage in viral or idiopathic pericarditis) or heart disease of any origin.

Chronic Pericarditis

In chronic pericardial diseases, there are no specific ECG signs. T negativity is common. A massive pericardial effusion can lead to peripheric low voltage. In *cardiac tamponade*, "electric alternans" might be present. However, today, this phenomenon is rarely seen, because therapy occurs earlier than it did decades ago, thanks to the echo. In *constrictive pericarditis*, atrial fibrillation is frequent, together with a general T negativity. Table 15.3 lists the etiologies of subacute/chronic pericarditis.

Table 15.3 Etiology in subacute/chronic pericarditis/chronic pericardial diseases

1. Common
   - Uremia (treated and untreated)
   - Neoplasias: lung, breast, melanoma, leukemia, Hodgkin's disease, lymphoma
   - Tuberculosis
   - Myxoedema
   - Delayed injury: postpericardiotomy syndrome

2. Rare
   - Infection: AIDS, inflammatory bowel disease, sarcoidosis, amyloidosis, amebiasis
   - Radiation
   - Autoimmune disorders: systemic lupus erythematodes, periarteritis nodosa, dermatomyositis, rheumatoid arthritis, scleroderma
   - Delayed injury: postmyocardial infarction syndrome (Dressler syndrome)
   - Primary tumors: sarcoma, mesothelioma
   - Chylopericardium
   - Pacemaker implantation

Chapter 16
Electrolyte Imbalance and Disturbances

Clinically important abnormalities of electrolytes more often involve potassium (K) than calcium (Ca). A pathologic cellular or serum level of natrium is not detectable in the electrocardiogram (ECG), as is also the case for hypomagnesemia, which is often combined with hypokalemia. Generally, the correlation between definitively pathologic electrolyte serum levels and the ECG is disappointingly poor (10%–30%). More important, severe or extreme electrolyte imbalance is detectable in the ECG up to 90%. The recognition of typical ECG patterns or arrhythmias may represent the first indication of a severe electrolyte disturbance. For instance, an extremely broad QRS may be attributable to hyperkalemia, and a ventricular tachycardia (VT) of the type torsade de pointes may indicate hypokalemia.

In many cases of electrolyte imbalance, the etiology is known in advance. Other causes of electrolyte imbalance can be found in a detailed checklist in my comprehensive book *The ECG*, Springer, 2004.

Hyperkalemia/Hyperpotassemia

Every physician is familiar with the typical tall and peaked, so-called *tented* T waves of hyperkalemia, generally present in mild or moderate hyperkalemia. Surprisingly, the ECG pattern in severe hyperkalemia is not as well known and is sometimes incorrectly interpreted. However, this ECG represents an urgent situation. It is characterized by extremely broad QRS complexes measuring up to 0.2 or even 0.26 s, with an atypical bundle-branch block pattern (ECGs 16.1 and 16.2). Additionally, a tall T wave is generally seen. Often, the p wave is not visible, thus imitating a ventricular rhythm (ECG 16.1). In fact, sinus rhythm is present, without visible sinusal p waves at the rate of the "assumed" ventricular rhythm because the potassium-induced "intoxication" of the atria inhibits a visible atrial depolarization. Severe hyperpotassemia is also responsible for the atypical ventricular aberration. Life-threatening arrhythmias can develop, such as VT and fibrillation or ventricular asystole. In rare cases, a marked ST elevation is present, mimicking acute myocardial injury, called *dialyzable injury*. ECG 16.3a–c illustrates the ECG patterns of a patient with terminal renal failure and severe hyperkalemia, regressing during hemodialysis.

M. Gertsch, *The ECG Manual: An Evidence-Based Approach*,
© Springer-Verlag London Limited 2009

ECG 16.1 Electrocardiogram (ECG) obtained from a 64-year-old woman with terminal renal failure. Hyperkalemia. ECG: probably sinus rhythm, with invisible p waves, rate 54 beats/min. Atypical right bundle-branch block pattern (QRS duration 0.16 s). Striking ST elevation in leads V_1 to V_3 (I, aVR, aVL) as sign of "dialyzable injury." K^+ 8.7 mmol/L

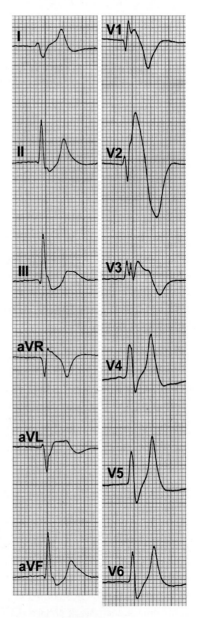

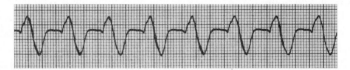

ECG 16.2 Electrocardiogram (ECG) obtained from a 44-year-old woman with Morbus Cushing after hypophysectomy, hypertension, diuretics containing amiloride. Hyperkalemia. ECG: monitor strip. Probable sinus rhythm with invisible p waves, rate 108 beats/min. Atypical left bundle-branch block pattern, QRS duration of approximately 0.18 s. Ventricular tachycardia of moderate rate is imitated. K^+ 9.4 mmol/L

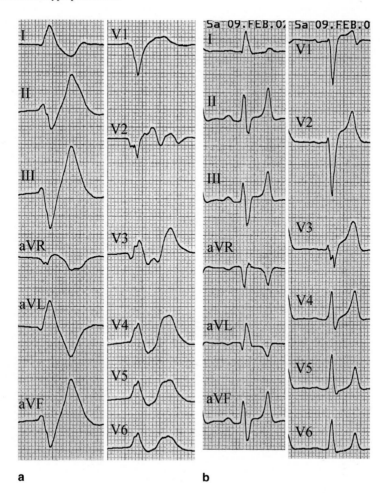

a   b

ECG 16.3 Electrocardiogram (ECG) obtained from a 60-year-old man. **a.** Terminal renal failure, hemodialysis (HD) three times weekly, for 2 years. The patient came 2 days too late for HD because of his birthday celebration. Hyperkalemia. ECG: probably sinus rhythm (SR) (without visible p waves), 58 beats/min. Very broad left bundle-branch block–like QRS (240 ms), bizarre broad T waves, concordant to QRS in V_3 to V_6. K^+ 8.97 mmol/L (Ca^{2+} 0.96 mmol/L). Therapy was immediate HD. **b.** After 30 min of HD, SR was 78 beats/min. Still slightly prolonged QRS duration, peaky and tall T waves, especially in the inferior leads. K^+ 5.87 mmol/L (Ca^{2+} 1.13 mmol/L)

ECG 16.3 (continued) **c.** After 60 min of HD, normal broad QRS, peaky T waves in several leads. K+ 5.90 mmol/L (!) (Ca^{2+} 1.19 mmol/L)

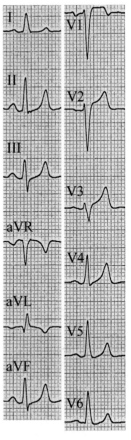

c

The ECG in moderate hyperkalemia shows the well-known tall, peaked, and symmetricoid ("tented") T waves, especially in the middle or lateral precordial leads (ECG 16.4), and less in the inferior frontal leads. Common etiologies of hyperkalemia are renal failure, hyperglycemia (diabetic ketoacidosis), drugs, and toxin(e)s. (See a detailed list in M. Gertsch, *The ECG*, Springer, 2004).

ECG 16.4 Electrocardiogram obtained from a 62-year-old man 2 days after intestinal operation. Hyperkalemia. Sinus rhythm, 86 beats/min. Normal QRS. Tall and peaky T waves in leads V_3 and V_4/V_5 (V_6). K^+ 5.8 mmol/L

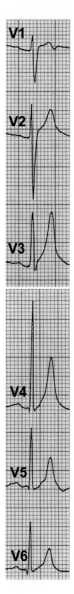

Hypokalemia (Hypopotassemia)

The ECG in severe hypokalemia is characterized by a fusion of the T wave with a prominent U wave (ECG 16.5). The QT interval cannot be measured, because the end of the T wave is not identifiable. The ST segment might or might not be depressed. ECG alterations similar to those attributable to hypokalemia are seen in patients under amiodarone, but in this case with a prominent U wave. Similar to the "true" (congenital) "long QT syndromes" (see Chapter 26), other conditions with TU fusion favor episodes of polymorphous VT of the type torsades de pointes (see Short Story). This type of VT has a high rate (between 160 and 300 beats/min) but

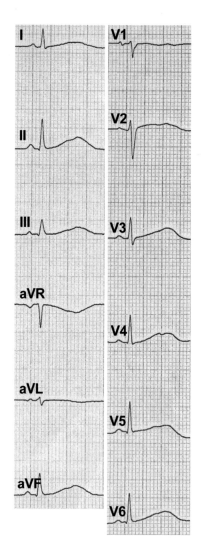

ECG 16.5 Electrocardiogram (ECG) obtained from a 53-year-old woman. Short syncope, antidepressants, and furosemide. Hypokalemia. ECG: almost complete TU fusion in all leads. No ST depression. K$^+$ 2.8 mmol/L. Holter ECG: short episodes of ventricular tachycardia type torsades de pointes

usually converts into sinus rhythm spontaneously. However, longer episodes lead to syncope or the tachycardia could degenerate into ventricular fibrillation. Hypokalemia is seen in conjunction with diarrhea, vomiting (inclusively anorexia) and after drugs, especially loop diuretics (see detailed list in M. Gertsch, *The ECG*, Springer). The Short Story demonstrates tremendous episodes of VT type torsade de pointes in a young woman with severe hypokalemia caused by bulimia.

Short Story

In March 2000, a 19-year-old woman with bulimia and irregular intake of diuretic drugs experienced several syncope episodes during the previous weeks with loss of consciousness up to 10 minutes. At entry into the hospital, the patient had no complaints, and body weight was normal. The ECG showed sinus bradycardia alternating with atrioventricular dissociation, at a rate of 40–45 beats/min (ECG 16.6a). The QTc (QTUc, respectively) was 0.56 s and there was a somewhat unusual fusion of the T wave with the U wave (ECG 16.6b). K^+ was 2.3 mmol/L (3.4–5.2), and Mg^+ 0.71 mmol/L (0.7–1.0). The patient was electrographically monitored, and K^+ and Mg^+ substitution was begun. After a short time, approximately 30 episodes of VT occurred, at a rate up to >300 beats/min, lasting from 4 to 22 seconds at maximum. In some ECG strips, torsades de pointes were identified (ECG 16.6c, ECG 16.6d), but in others showed a monomorphic VT with the pattern of ventricular flutter (ECG 16.6e). The patient became dizzy at times but lost consciousness only rarely, for a few seconds. Defibrillation was not necessary. After 4 hours, the VT episodes stopped. The following day, K^+ was within normal limits, the QTUc was still prolonged, and episodes of bradycardiac atrioventricular dissociation persisted. K^+ was given orally and 3 days later the patient could be dismissed with a normal ECG (sinus rhythm 72 beats/min, QTUc 0.46 s) and a K^+ serum level of 4.8 mmol/l. An ambulant psychiatric therapy was organized.

Severe hypokalemia can represent a dangerous condition. Hypomagnesemia or a preexisting prolonged QT (e.g., caused by drugs) favors the development of torsades de pointes VT. The treating physicians were very happy about the favorable outcome in this young woman, considering the episodes of VT at rates up to 360 beats/min.

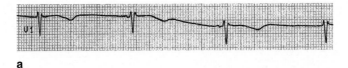

a

ECG 16.6 Electrocardiogram (ECG) obtained from the 19-year-old woman described in the Short Story. Hypokalemia **a**. (Rhythm strip, V_1) Bradycardic isorhythmic atrioventricular dissociation, rate 42 beats/min

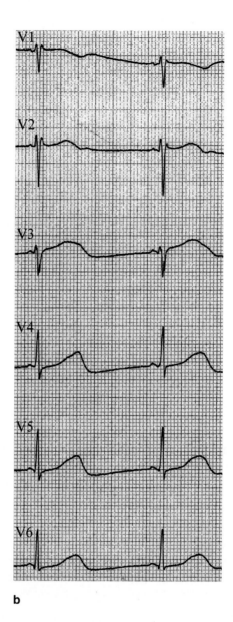

b

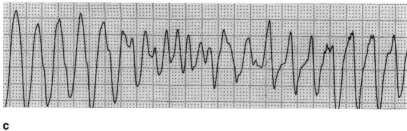

c

ECG 16.6. (continued) **b.** Completely fused T and U waves. QT(U) 620 ms. QT(U)c 521 ms. Incomplete right bundle-branch block. **c.** (Rhythm strip) Ventricular tachycardia (VT) of the type torsades de pointes, rate >300 beats/min

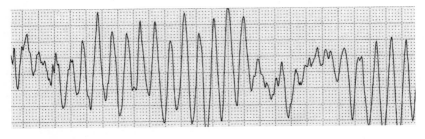

d

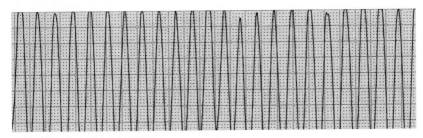

e

ECG 16.6 (continued) **d.** (Rhythm strip) VT of the type torsades de pointes, maximal instantaneous rate up to 360 beats/min. **e.** (Rhythm strip) Almost regular VT with morphology of ventricular
flutter, rate approximately 220 beats/min

Hypercalcemia

In moderate to severe hypercalcemia, the ECG is characterized by a shortened QT
interval, always at the expense of the ST segment that is shortened or even absent
(ECGs 16.7). Although the ECG pattern is striking and observance of the ECG
computer print, which indicates QTc time, often provides the diagnosis, this condition is often overlooked even by experienced ECG readers for the following
reasons:

1. The pattern is rare.
2. The ECG looks otherwise normal.
3. Experienced ECG readers sometimes become overconfident.

Hypercalcemia can be found in patients with primary or secondary hyperparathyroidism, tumors with or without metastases, acute and chronic renal
failure, and other conditions (see detailed list in M. Gertsch, *The ECG*,
Springer, 2004).

ECG 16.7 Electrocardiogram (ECG) obtained from a
47-year-old man with primary hyperparathyroidism.
Hypercalcemia. ECG: sinus rhythm 62 beats/min. Only
slightly reduced QT interval (368 ms, QTc 376 ms), but
visually "absent" ST segment. Ca^{2+} 2.88 mmol/L
(normal up to 2.5)

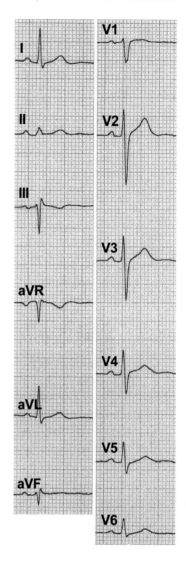

Hypocalcemia

Hypocalcemia is also a rare finding. In contrast to hypercalcemia, a prolonged ST
segment is found in the ECG, with a consecutive prolonged QT interval (ECG
16.8). Isolated hypocalcemia is caused by hypoalbuminemia and disturbances in
parathormone and vitamin D metabolism, generally in patients with chronic renal
disease (see detailed list in M. Gertsch, *The ECG*, Springer, 2004). Interestingly,
hypocalcemia never provokes VT of the torsade de pointes type, although the QT
interval is also prolonged as in hypokalemia.

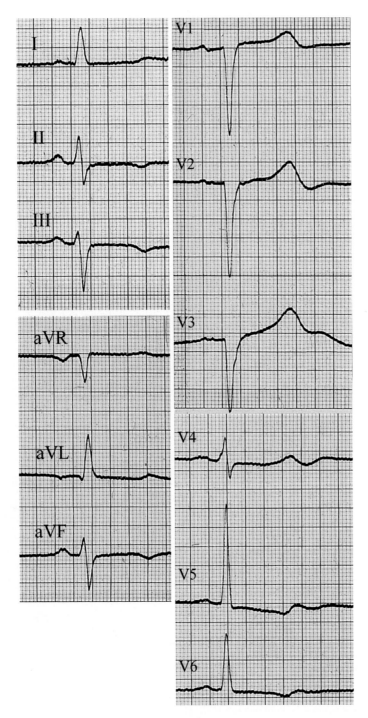

ECG 16.8 Electrocardiogram (ECG) obtained from a 73-year-old woman. Hypocalcemia. ECG (50 mm/s): prolonged QT interval, with prolonged ST segment and "late" T wave

The combination of hypocalcemia and hyperkalemia is mainly seen in patients with chronic renal failure. The ECG shows a prolonged ST segment with QT lengthening and tall and somewhat peaked T waves (ECG 16.9).

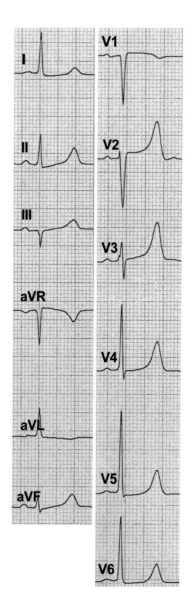

ECG 16.9 Electrocardiogram (ECG) obtained from a 67-year-old woman with chronic renal failure. Hyperkalemia plus hypocalcemia. ECG: sinus rhythm, 63 beats/min. QT interval 497 ms, QTc 510 ms. Tall and peaky T waves in V_2 to V_6 (II, aVF). No detectable U wave. K^+ 6.2 mmol/L; Ca^{2+} 1.4 mmol/L

Therapy for Severe Hyperkalemia

The fast recognition of the ECG pattern in severe hyperkalemia allows a rapid and simple therapy: 10 mL of slowly administered intravenous calcium gluconate normalizes the cellular membrane potential and consecutively the ECG within minutes. Further therapy depends on the underlying disease, usually renal insufficiency or hyperglycemia.

Therapy for Severe Hypokalemia

Therapy consists of potassium substitution which is generally completed by magnesium substitution. Hypomagnesemia, not detectable in the ECG, often accompanies hypokalemia, especially when the potassium deficit is caused by diuretic drugs. A transient pacemaker may be useful.

Chapter 17
Alterations of Repolarization

Pathologic negative T waves represent the most frequent isolated deformations of ventricular repolarization. However, T wave alterations that are not related to pathologic QRS complexes are very nonspecific. The alterations of the ST segment are rarer and somewhat more specific.

ST Segment

ST Elevation

Acute myocardial infarction represents the most important clinical form of ST elevation, often with a voltage of ≥ 3 mm. This value is reached only in some other, rare conditions such as Prinzmetal's angina, early repolarization, the Brugada syndrome, and as a mirror image in left ventricular hypertrophy (LVH)/overload, in this case in lead V_2. In acute pericarditis, ST elevation rarely exceeds 2 mm.

ST elevation in limb leads produces ST depression in the opposite leads, as mirror images (e.g., ST elevation in aVL → ST depression in aVF/III; ST elevation in III/aVF → ST depression in aVL). In acute posterior myocardial infarction, we see the primary ST elevation in the additional leads V_7 to V_9, as ST depression V (mirror image) V in leads (V_1) V_2/V_3 (V_4). The differential diagnosis of isolated ST elevation is relatively small (Table 17.1).

ST Depression

The most important clinical ST depression occurs during exercise test (in leads V_4 to V_6) as a marker of ischemia. ST depression at rest is relatively rare in pure ischemia. As mentioned above, significant ST depression in leads V_2/V_3 (V_1) corresponds to a mirror image of acute posterior myocardial infarction but never to isolated subendocardial anteroseptal ischemia, which cannot be identified in the electrocardiogram (ECG).

M. Gertsch, *The ECG Manual: An Evidence-Based Approach*,
© Springer-Verlag London Limited 2009

Table 17.1 Differential diagnosis of ST elevation

Condition	Typical signs
Acute myocardial infarction (AMI)	ST arising from the R wave
	Amplitude 2–10 mm
	Frontal ST vector: inferior AMI
	approximately +90°; anterior AMI
	approximately +40°
	Evolution to Q wave infarction
Prinzmetal's angina	Morphology and amplitude as in
	AMI. Regression within 20 min
	Reversible within 15–20 min
Early repolarization	ST, arising from the R or S wave
	Amplitude 1–5 mm
	No evolution. Healthy often young people
Vagotonia	Amplitude up to 4 mm in leads V_2/V_3
	Mostly in sinus bradycardia
Pericarditis stage 2	ST mostly arising from the S wave
	Amplitude <2 mm
	Frontal ST vector approximately
	+70° (ST elevation in I *and* aVF!)
	Evolution: No pathologic Q wave!
Mirror image of left	Amplitude up to 4 mm in leads V_2/V_3
ventricular overload	High amplitude mostly associated
	with left ventricular hypertrophy
Brugada syndrome	Amplitude up to 3 mm in V_2, less in V_1/V_3
	Combined with the pattern of incomplete
	right bundle-branch block
	Suppressed by class I antiarrhythmic drugs
Other rare conditions	

Note: A simplified "rule" implies that in AMI the elevated ST segment arises from the R wave, whereas in acute pericarditis (stage 2), the elevated ST segment arises from the S wave. This rule is valid in only about 90% of cases for AMI, and in about 80% for pericarditis.

In the ECG at rest, ST depression in leads V_5/V_6 (and I/aVL), associated with asymmetric negative T waves in the same leads, is generally attributable to left ventricular (LV) overload, with or without LVH. In this case, a mirror image in leads V_1/V_2 is often observed. Digitalis often leads to mild, approximately 1 mm ST depression, with a typical tub-like configuration. Slight ST depression, up to 1 mm, is found in many conditions and is therefore nonspecific.

T Wave

T Negativity

Negative asymmetric T waves are a frequent normal finding in several limb leads (Table 17.2). In these conditions, T negativity is related to the frontal QRS axis ($\mathring{A}QRS_F$). In vertical $\mathring{A}QRS_F$, there is T negativity in III, aVF(II); in left $\mathring{A}QRS_F$, T negativity in aVL.

Table 17.2 Differential diagnosis of T negativity

Classical non-Q infarction
Ischemia without infarction
Ventricular overload
Normal variants
Syndrome X
Pericarditis (stages 3 and 4)
Myocarditis
Severe anemia
Funnel chest
Upright position
Drugs
Pancreatitis
Innumerable other diseases and conditions*

*Negative T waves in some precordial leads are not
only encountered in ischemia, but also in countless
other conditions, too numerous to list.

A negative T wave in lead I is usually pathologic. In the precordial leads, a negative T wave is only found in lead V_1 in normal hearts. As an exception, occasionally a negative T wave can be present in leads V_2 and V_3 in healthy men up to age 25 and in healthy women up to age 35. However, in the presence of T negativity in leads V_2/V_3, an abnormality of the right ventricle should be considered (e.g., atrial septal defect, pulmonary embolism, arrhythmogenic right ventricle).

Negative T waves resulting from ischemia are called *primary negative T waves* and secondary T waves from ventricular hypertrophy are called *secondary negative T waves*. In ischemia, the negative T wave is generally symmetric (ECG 17.1), whereas in LV overload, which is often associated with LVH, the negative T wave is generally asymmetric (ECG 17.2). However, this rule is not reliable. For instance, negative symmetric T waves are also found in pericarditis (stages 3 and 4), hypertrophic cardiomyopathy, and other diseases. The differential diagnosis of asymmetric negative T waves is even more extensive and includes normal hearts, inflammations, general diseases, drug effects, and so on. Moreover, asymmetric T waves may have a symmetric aspect at their apex. It would be incongruous to diagnose LV overload/LVH *and* ischemia, based on this pattern.

T Positivity

Positive T waves are rarely pathologic. Abnormally tall and symmetroid T waves are seen in moderate hyperkalemia. The same T morphology, however, is observed in the earliest stage of myocardial infarction, lasting only minutes. The differential diagnosis for tall T waves in V_2/V_3 is normal variants, especially in sinus bradycardia.

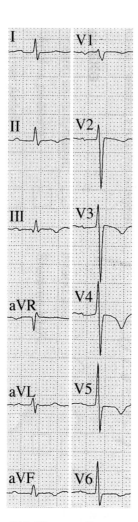

ECG 17.1 Electrocardiogram (ECG) obtained from a 70-year-old man with coronary heart disease and pulmonary emphysema. Typical chest pain occurred 20 minutes before the ECG. ECG: symmetric negative T waves in leads V_2 to V_6. Note also peripheral near low voltage and atrioventricular block 1°. Coro: proximal 90% stenosis of the left anterior descending coronary artery. Minimal apical hypokinesia

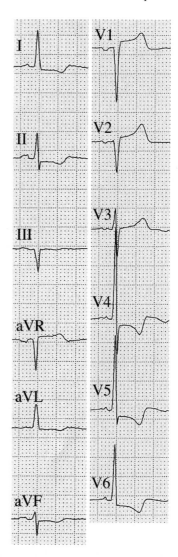

ECG 17.2 Electrocardiogram (ECG) obtained from a 52-year-old woman with hypertension and combined aortic valve disease. Normal coronary arteries. ECG: high R voltage in leads V_4 to V_6. ST depression and negative asymmetric T waves in I, II, aVL, aVF, and V_4 to V_6 (in V_4 the T wave is nearly symmetric)

Short Story/Case Report

In November 1998, a 65-year-old man with a history of stable angina felt a sudden strong typical chest pain during routine ECG registration. The skilled nurse was struck by the tall symmetric T waves in leads V_2/V_3 (ECG 17.3) and referred the patient immediately to the coronary care unit. There, the patient developed an acute anterior infarction with a typical ECG within 20 minutes. Coronary angiography was performed 50 minutes after the onset of pain. The proximal left anterior descending coronary artery was closed. The results of percutaneous coronary transluminal angioplasty and stenting were excellent. The akinetic apical zone regressed to a slight hypokinesia.

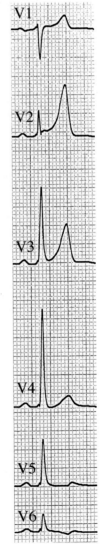

ECG 17.3 Electrocardiogram obtained from a 65-year-old man, described in the Short Story, with high symmetric T waves with slight ST elevation in leads V_2/V_3. Note that very similar T waves in these leads are seen as normal variants

Giant Negative T Waves

Giant negative T waves, with an amplitude of 5–15 mm, are rare. In combination with LVH, they are found in some cases of hypertension, in hypertrophic cardiomyopathy, and in many patients with apical hypertrophy, a very rare disease. Isolated giant negative T waves, which lack QRS alterations, are observed in the classical non–Q wave infarction pattern, in combination with cerebral diseases, in some cases of postpacing T negativity (Chatterjee phenomenon), and after pulmonary edema. They are also seen with the so-called global T wave inversion, which is predominantly found in women and associated with a good prognosis.

Giant negative T waves with an obvious or even excessive QT prolongation represent a rare ECG pattern, formerly called *postsyncopal bradycardia syndrome*. However, the pattern can arise without a previous syncope and be combined with normocardia. In about half of the cases, a cerebral disease such as subarachnoidal hemorrhage, a cerebral insult, or an epileptic attack precedes the appearance of the ECG alteration. In the other 50%, the etiology remains unclear.

Patterns with Prolonged or Shortened QT Duration

Repolarization is altered per se in the presence of prolonged or shortened QT. In the congenital "long QT syndrome"—with deafness referred to as Jervell and Lange-Nielsen syndrome, without deafness Romano-Ward syndrome—as well as in the acquired long QT syndrome, often the result of hypokalemia and antiarrhythmic drugs, the ST segment is isoelectric but can show slight depression or even elevation. The T wave is generally fused with the U wave (see Chapter 16). The recently discovered congenital "short QT syndrome" is extremely rare.

Chapter 18
Atrial Premature Beats

Atrial premature beats (APBs) are slightly less frequent than ventricular premature beats (VPBs) but much more frequent than supraventricular premature beats arising in the atrioventricular (AV) junction. Often, APBs are not associated with heart disease. In up to 64% of healthy young individuals, some APBs are found in an ambulatory electrocardiogram (Holter ECG), and in most cases without symptoms.

APBs are characterized by premature onset and a deformed p wave, indicating origin of a mostly right atrial "focus," distant from the sinus node (ECG 18.1). A focus in the low right atrium, near the coronary sinus, leads to negative p waves in the inferior leads aVF, III (and II). The short PQ interval may be equal or slightly longer (>0.12 s) as in an AV junction beat. ECG 18.2 shows an example of ectopic atrial rhythm with negative p waves inferiorly and in leads V_2 to V_6 in an older patient with right ventricular hypertrophy. A negative p wave in I, aVL, and V_6/V_5 may be attributable to either ectopic right or left atrial origin, but only the latter is associated with a positive p wave in lead V_1.

As in VPBs, prematurity is not constant. In contrast to VPBs, the pause after the APB usually does not show full compensation (also in VPBs compensation is not always complete). If the p wave falls into the T wave of the preceding cardiac cycle, it can be difficult to identify. Whereas the first APB in ECG 18.3 (with a short PQ interval and negative p waves in V_3 to V_6) is clearly visible, the second, very early APB is only detectable by a peak on the T wave in V_1 (and V_2), because of a superimposed p wave. There is aberration with a right bundle-branch block pattern. The last beat may be interpreted as postextrasystolic atrial escape, from the same focus as the first APB. After early APBs, aberration (ECG 18.3) or AV block 1° can be observed. In aberration of early APBs, right bundle-branch block is more frequent than left bundle-branch block. If the APB occurs very early, it may be completely AV blocked (ECG 18.4). In these cases, the false diagnosis of sinuatrial block is occasionally made. If an APB falls in the potentially vulnerable phase of the repolarization of the preceding atrial beat ("p on Ta"), it may induce atrial fibrillation.

Atrial bigeminy is rare; salvos of APBs are occasionally observed. In contrast to short episodes of atrial tachycardia, the rhythm is irregular and can lead to diagnostic difficulties (see Short Story).

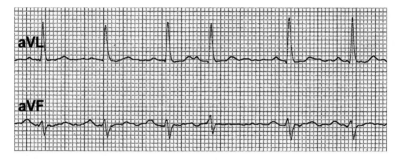

ECG 18.1 Atrial premature beat (leads aVL/aVF)

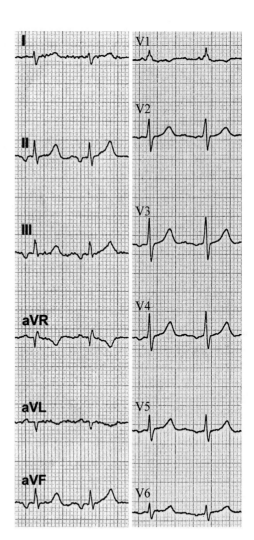

ECG 18.2 Electrocardiogram obtained from a 67-year-old man with right ventricular hypertrophy caused by chronic obstructive pneumopathy. Because the PQ interval is approximately 0.12 s, the origin of the rhythm might be localized to the inferior portion of the right atrium or to the atrioventricular junction

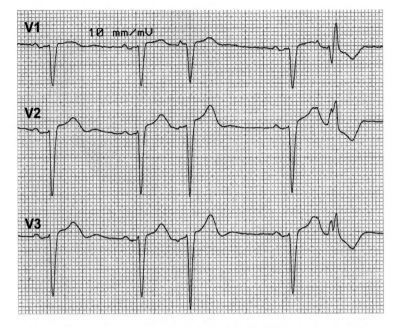

ECG 18.3 Two atrial premature beats with different coupling intervals. The second one, with a short coupling interval, shows right bundle-branch block aberration

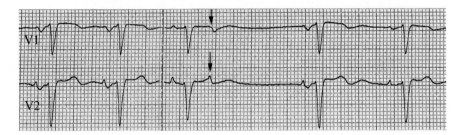

ECG 18.4 Atrioventricular blocked atrial premature beat (APB). The APB occurs very early and is blocked. The previous beat is a normal sinus beat; the p wave is deformed by an artifact

Short Story/Case Report

Some years ago, a 62-year-old specialist with a good reputation in internal medicine told the author that, in his mind, the ECG is a "method for the foxes" that never helped him with a correct diagnosis. The author warmly congratulated him for his modern concept. In October 2000, the author received a long letter from this specialist. An ECG with a rhythm strip was enclosed (ECG 18.5). The

39-year-old patient, the physician's *daughter*, suffered from tachycardic palpitations, associated with vertigo and near syncope. The physician's rhythm diagnosis was: basically normal ECG. Sinus arrhythmia, atypical AV reentry tachycardia with AV dissociation, and perhaps an AV block. The author was very eager to analyze such an unusual arrhythmia. His diagnosis was: basically normal ECG. APBs in salvos up to 12 beats, at a rate about 150 beats/min. Proposition: atenolol (25 or 12.5 mg). Looking for infectious parameters. Echo/Doppler. Holter ECG. Exercise ECG. Thereafter, decision about definitive therapy. The conclusion: The ECG may suddenly become important when a near relative shows symptoms.

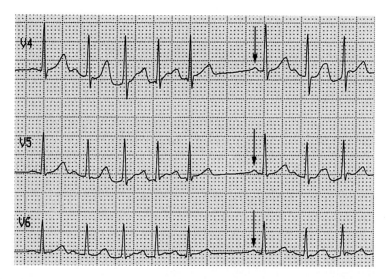

ECG 18.5 Electrocardiogram (ECG) obtained from a 39-year-old woman, described in the Short Story. ECG (leads V$_4$ to V$_6$): only one sinusoidal beat (↓), runs of atrial premature beats, maximal instantaneous rate 165 beats/min

Chapter 19
Atrial Tachycardias (Without Atrial Flutter/Fibrillation)

Atrial tachycardias are not frequent if atrial fibrillation and atrial flutter are excluded (see corresponding chapters). The types of atrial tachycardia differ in regard to morphology of the p wave, atrial rate, atrioventricular (AV) conduction, duration of the arrhythmia, hemodynamic consequences, electrophysiologic mechanism, and etiology.

In all atrial tachycardias, the p waves precede the QRS complex, but p morphology is different from sinusal p waves. Most atrial tachycardias are regular. Based on clinical significance, atrial tachycardias can be classified as listed in the following text.

"Salvos" of Atrial Premature Beats

The episodes of atrial premature beats (APBs) (often 3–5 beats) are generally of moderate rate (110–150 beats/min) and often without symptoms. ECG 19.1 shows a longer episode of 8 beats.

Ectopic (Focal) Atrial Tachycardia

Ectopic (focal) atrial tachycardia is attributed to enhanced automaticity of an ectopic atrial focus. The morphology of the p waves depends on the localization of the ectopic center. P is negative or positive in the inferior leads III and aVF. Often, this regular tachycardia is of short duration (up to 30s), with a rate generally between 110 and 150 beats/min (ECG 19.2). Therefore, the tachycardia is called benign slow atrial tachycardia. Rates up to 180 beats/min are rare. The rare incessant form, with duration of weeks or months, is often associated with organic heart disease but the tachycardia itself can lead to ventricular dilatation and heart failure, which is at least partially reversible after catheter-ablation. It is especially seen in young people.

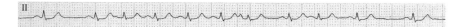

ECG 19.1 Electrocardiogram obtained from a 29-year-old woman. Run of 8 atrial premature beats with a moderate rate, irregular

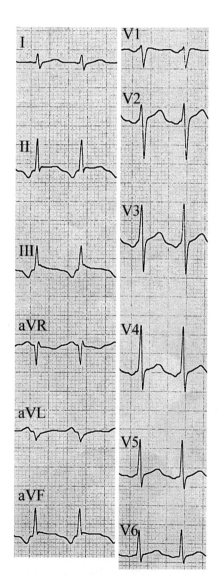

ECG 19.2 Electrocardiogram (ECG) obtained from a 45-year-old healthy man with no symptoms. ECG: atrial tachycardia of 127 beats/ min. Negative p waves in inferior limb leads and V_1 to V_5 (V_6). PQ 0.1 s. Note ST elevation, caused by inverse atrial repolarization

At the beginning of the tachycardia, aberrant conduction can be present (mainly right bundle-branch block) that disappears after several beats, at the same rate. A longer tachycardia often shows some changes in the rate. Alterations of the repolarization are common and can persist for hours after conversion of the tachycardia. Short episodes are harmless and generally occur in healthy individuals. Long episodes (incessant form) are more often associated with organic heart disease. Vagal maneuvers do not influence the atrial rate, but can induce AV block 2°. Adenosine is sometimes successful. In problematic cases, catheter ablation is the best therapy.

Atrial Reentry Tachycardia

The reentry circuit consists of two distinct intraatrial functional pathways. Again, the p wave is different from a sinusal p and may be positive or negative in III and aVF. The tachycardia is introduced by an APB. In contrast to the focal type, p wave morphology often changes, according to variations within the circuit. Moreover, at the beginning of the tachycardia, an increase of the rate can be observed (so-called "warming up effect"). Generally, the rate is higher than in ectopic atrial tachycardia and can reach 240 beats/min. The incidence is about 6% in patients with paroxysmal supraventricular tachycardias, studied invasively. Atrial reentry tachycardia is found in patients with otherwise healthy hearts but also in those with congenital and other heart diseases. Vagal maneuvers and adenosine are rarely successful. ECG 19.3 demonstrates that drug conversion with adenosine may also provoke a tremble in the treating physician's heart.

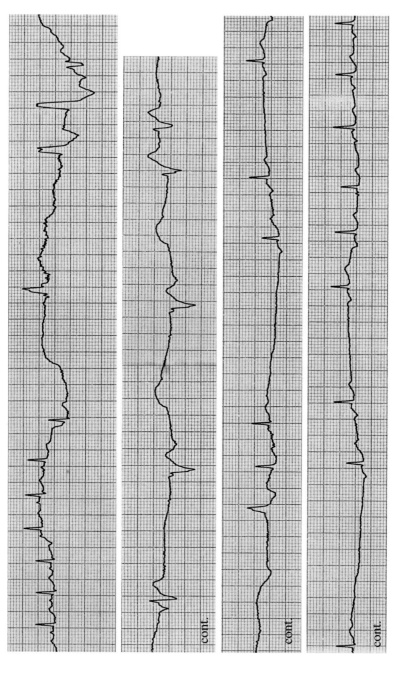

ECG 19.3 Electrocardiogram obtained from a 52-year-old man who experienced several episodes of rapid palpitations lasting minutes to 2 hours. Rarely vertigo. Otherwise healthy heart. Continuous rhythm-strip (monitor lead): atrial tachycardia (electrophysiologic investigation—atrial reentry tachycardia) at 160 beats/min. Conversion with 6 mg of intravenous adenosine. Note several episodes of significant bradycardia with pauses up to 2.5 s, as a result of sinus standstill or sinoatrial block, with ventricular and atrial escape beats. Finally, ectopic atrial rhythm

Repetitive Paroxysmal Atrial Tachycardia

This arrhythmia is very rare. It is defined by excessively frequent paroxysms of a slightly irregular atrial tachycardia with a rate of 130–150 beats/min. A more or less incessant tachycardia may be present, frequently interrupted by some sinus beats. The therapy depends on the symptoms and the underlying heart disease.

Paroxysmal Atrial Tachycardia with Atrioventricular Block

Atrial tachycardia rarely show an AV block 1°. The term "atrial tachycardia with block" is reserved for the presence of AV block 2° (and, extremely rare, AV block 3°). The mechanism of tachycardia is probably an "ectopic focus." The rate is often between 150 and 200 beats/min, with a range from 110 to 240 beats/min. Usually, AV block 2:1 is present (ECG 19.4), rarely with superimposed Wenckebach phenomenon

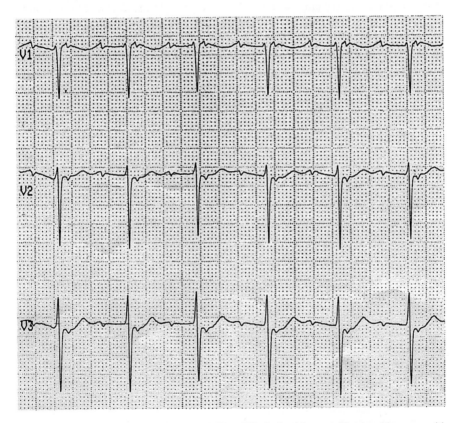

ECG 19.4 Electrocardiogram (ECG) (leads V_1 to V_3) obtained from an 85-year-old woman with coronary and hypertensive heart disease. Mild renal failure (creatinine 130 mmol/L, creatinine clearance not known). Serum digoxin level 5.7 mmol/L. ECG: atrial tachycardia, 156 beats/min, with 2:1 atrioventricular (AV) block. The conducted beats show AV block 1°. Rare ventricular premature beats and relatively mild ST depression in V_3 to V_6 (not shown). Normalization of the rhythm within 7 days (over Wenckebach and AV block 1°)

(leading to irregularity of the ventricular action) or AV block 3:1. Often, the atrial rhythm is slightly irregular. Occasionally, an alternating slight "regular irregularity" is found: the (AV blocked) p wave after the QRS shows a shorter distance to the previous (conducted) p than to the following (again conducted) p wave. The differentiation between the arrhythmia and atrial flutter with 2:1 AV block, especially of type 2 (where "saw-tooth" waves are lacking, with a preserved isoelectric line between the flutter waves) is often not possible. However, the differentiation is clinically important in *one condition*: In atrial flutter, digitalis is often helpful for slowing the ventricular rate. If atrial tachycardia with AV block is the result of digitalis intoxication, digitalis is obsolete.

Left Atrial Tachycardia

This arrhythmia is very rare. Because of a possible high rate of 150–200 beats/min, it can cause severe symptoms. The electrocardiogram (ECG) is characterized by negative p waves in lead I and often in aVL, and by positive p waves in lead V_1 (ECG 19.5). Mirowski's ancient criteria have been modified because a similar p morphology can be observed in cases with ectopic *right* atrial tachycardia, but with a biphasic p wave in lead V_1. The reason for the positive p wave in lead V_1 in left atrial rhythm is an atypical activation of both atria, with both vectors oriented anteriorly. A 100% differentiation between right and left atrial origin is necessary, of course, if ablation therapy is taken into consideration.

ECG 19.5 Electrocardiogram (ECG) obtained from a 54-year-old woman with left atrial tachycardia. Palpitations for years. Supraventricular tachycardia rate 125 beats/min. Note the negative p waves in leads I, II, and V_2 to V_6, and the high positive p wave in V_1. Electrophysiologic investigation: focus in the proximal right lower lung vein. Ablation. (ECG courtesy of Reto Candinas.)

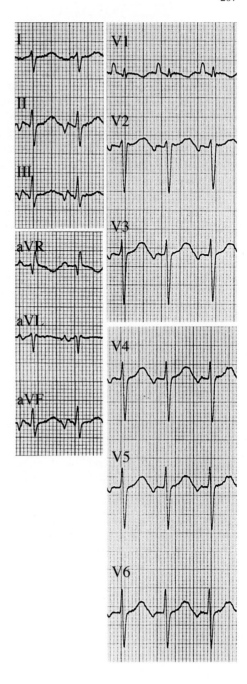

Multifocal Atrial Tachycardia (Chaotic Atrial Tachycardia)

Multifocal atrial tachycardia, also referred to as *chaotic atrial tachycardia* or *chaotic atrial mechanism*, is also very rare. The rate is approximately 110–150 beats/min, but sometimes less than 100 beats/min, at which point it is correctly called chaotic atrial mechanism (ECG 19.6). It is defined as: 1. at least three, often more than 10, different p morphologies in one lead; and 2. variable P-P, R-R, and PQ intervals. Because the absence of a dominant atrial center is also mandatory, *sinus rhythm with salvos of APBs* should *not* be misdiagnosed as multifocal/chaotic atrial tachycardia/mechanism.

AV block 1° can occur in some beats, as well as singular AV junction escape beats. The arrhythmia lasts for minutes up to days. It can change to atrial flutter or atrial fibrillation, but this has been exceptional in our experience. Multifocal atrial tachycardia has generally moderate hemodynamic consequences. Its bad prognosis is based on the frequent association with severe chronic obstructive pulmonary disease. In this context, up to 50% of the patients die within 6 months of the underlying disease. Diabetes, hypertensive heart disease, and hypokalemia are rarely associated with the arrhythmia.

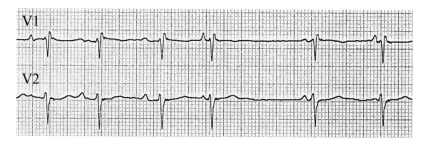

ECG 19.6 Electrocardiogram (ECG) obtained from a 64-year-old man with coronary artery disease. ECG (leads V_1/V_2): chaotic atrial rhythm, instantaneous rate 50–107 beats/min. Note the "absolute ventricular arrhythmia," the six different p waves in six cycles and the varying PQ intervals

Closing Remark

Recently, a new, not yet definitive, nomenclature of atrial tachycardias, atrial flutter inclusively, has been proposed (see Chapter 20).

Chapter 20
Atrial Flutter

Atrial flutter is 8 times rarer than atrial fibrillation, but increases to approximately 15 times in elderly patients. The arrhythmia may last for several beats, several minutes, hours, months, or even years. Symptoms preferentially depend on ventricular rate, which is determined by atrioventricular conduction. The etiology of atrial flutter is as manifold as that of atrial fibrillation.

The (atrial) rate of atrial flutter is between 230 and 330 beats/min, often between 260 and 300 beats/min, and is stable in an individual patient. Atrial impulses are frequently blocked within the atrioventricular (AV) node in a 2:1 mode (2:1 AV block), resulting in a ventricular rate of approximately 130–150 beats/min. Atrial rate is slowed by a dilated right atrium and an excessive intraatrial conduction disturbance. Drugs such as amiodarone will decrease the rate to less than 200 beats/min. Preexisting or rate-dependent right bundle-branch block (or rarely left bundle-branch block) might be present, masking the flutter waves and mimicking ventricular tachycardia at a first glance. A tachycardia with small or broad QRS, especially with right bundle-branch block configuration, at a rate of 130–160 beats/min, represents atrial flutter in approximately 70% of the cases (ECG 20.1).

Morphologic Types of Atrial Flutter

There are two principal types of atrial flutter, which are discussed below. For a recently published detailed nomenclature, see Table 20.1.

Common Type

The common type, type 1, accounts for 85% of cases of atrial flutter. Typical flutter waves show a sawtooth or picket fence appearance in leads III and aVF (and II), where the isoelectric line can no longer be identified, and flutter waves or p-like waves in some other leads are clearly visible in V_1 (ECGs 20.2 and 20.3). Often, the ventricular response is irregular, because of varying 2° AV block (2:1 to 4:1

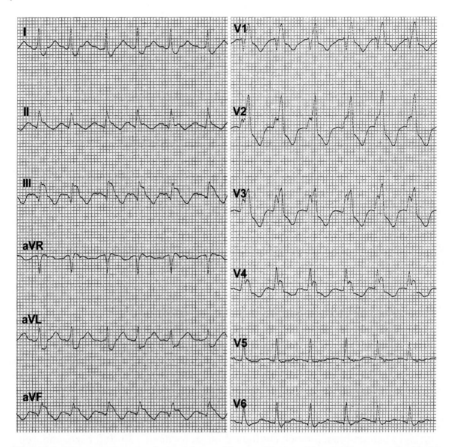

ECG 20.1 Electrocardiogram obtained from a 69-year-old man with atrial flutter type 1 with 2:1 (or 3:1) atrioventricular block and right bundle-branch block. Atrial rate 270 beats/min; ventricular rate 135 beats/min or fewer. The "sawtooth" flutter waves (inferiorly) are partially hidden within the negative T waves and the QRS complex. Note that the QRS complex in V_5 appears to be small, because the terminal part of QRS is almost isoelectric

Table 20.1 New nomenclature of atrial flutter

Typical flutter (formerly type 1 flutter) electrocardiogram: sawtooth/picket fence appearance
Reverse typical flutter (formerly type 2 flutter)
Lesion macroreentrant tachycardia ("incisional" flutter)
Lower loop flutter
Double wave reentry
Right atrial free wall macroreentry without atriotomy
Left atrial macroreentrant tachycardia (primary circuit in the left atrium)

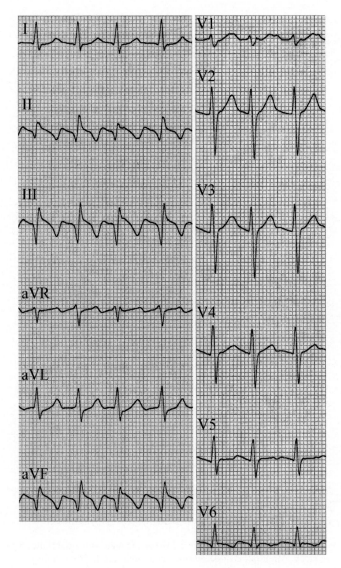

ECG 20.2 Electrocardiogram obtained from a 53-year-old man with atrial flutter type 1 with 1:2 atrioventricular (AV) conduction (2:1 AV block). Atrial rate 270 beats/min. Every other flutter wave is superimposed on the negative T waves in leads III/aVF/II, because of three previous inferior myocardial infarctions (see Q waves in these leads)

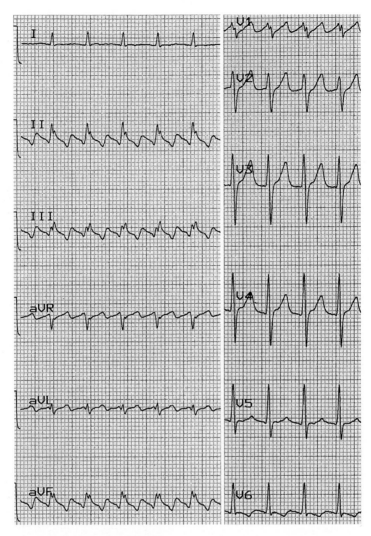

ECG 20.3 Electrocardiogram obtained from a 73-year-old man with atrial flutter type 1 with 2:1 atrioventricular block. Atrial rate 314 beats/min; ventricular rate 157 beats/min

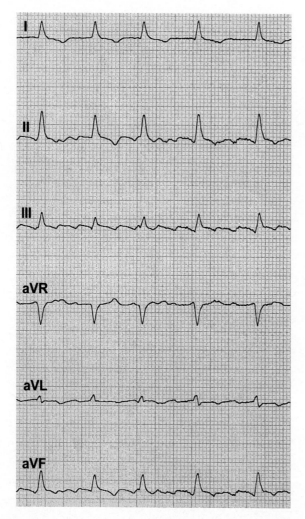

ECG 20.4 Electrocardiogram obtained from a 73-year-old man with atrial flutter type 1 (saw-tooth pattern only minimal; see lead III) with atrioventricular block 2:1 or 3:1, with superimposed Wenckebach phenomenon (interval between flutter waves and QRS changing). Atrial rate 276 beats/min. Left ventricular hypertrophy and left ventricular overload

or higher), sometimes with a superimposed Wenckebach mechanism (ECG 20.4), occasionally mimicking absolute arrhythmia as in atrial fibrillation. However, in a longer rhythm strip, a "regular irregularity" can be recognized in all cases, which could also indicate atrial flutter with changing AV conduction if the flutter waves cannot be identified (ECG 20.5).

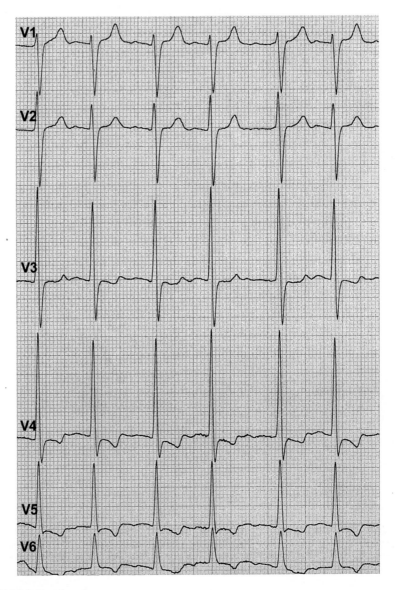

ECG 20.4 (continued)

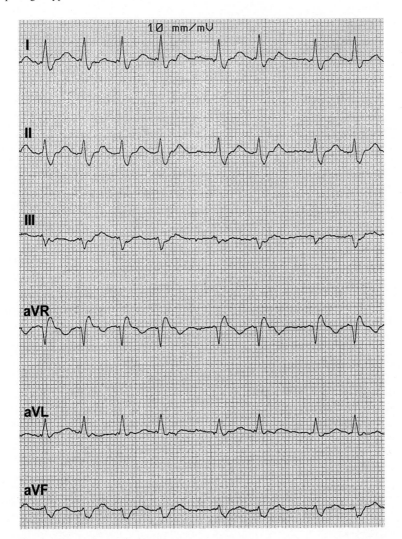

ECG 20.5 Atrial flutter without clearly detectable flutter waves in a patient with right bundle-branch block. The diagnosis is made on the basis of "regular irregularity," corresponding to 2:1 or 3:1 atrio-ventricular block. Flutter rate corresponds to double the instantaneous rate of the small R-R intervals = 284 beats/min

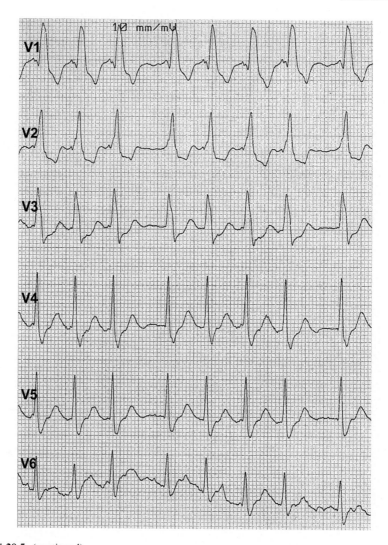

ECG 20.5 (continued)

A conduction rate of 1:1 is rare, but important. It can occur in children, but also in adults during sympathetic stimulation, e.g., during exercise (see ECG 20.6a; for 2:1 AV block after exercise, see ECG 20.6b), in the early phase of quinidine therapy, and in patients with preexcitation, as in Wolff-Parkinson-White syndrome. A ventricular response of approximately 300 beats/min is a dangerous condition. Moreover, ventricular fibrillation can develop.

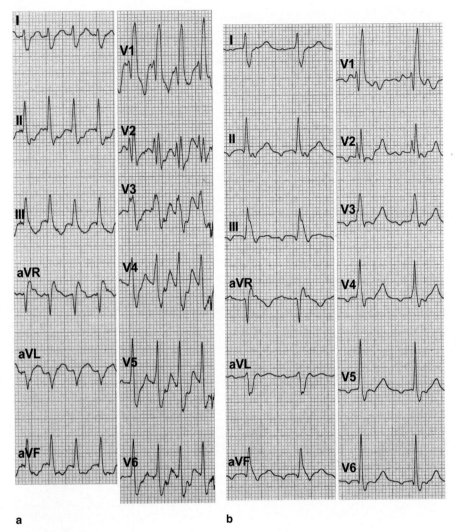

a   b

ECG 20.6 Electrocardiograms obtained from a 47-year-old man. **a.** Tetralogy of Fallot, operated at the age of 26 years. Atrial flutter with 1:1 conduction during exercise (9 MET), ventricular rate 205 beats/min. Right bundle-branch block. The low atrial rate is caused by an excessively dilated right atrium. **b.** The patient at rest. Atrial flutter type 1 with atrioventricular block 2° 2:1. Atrial rate 204 beats/min

Uncommon Type

The uncommon type, type 2, is also called reversed type 1, and accounts for 15% of the cases of atrial flutter. Its diagnosis can be difficult because the sawtooth configuration is lacking. Type 2 flutter waves are p wave-like in all leads, and positive in leads III and aVF, with a relatively preserved isoelectric line (ECG 20.7). The

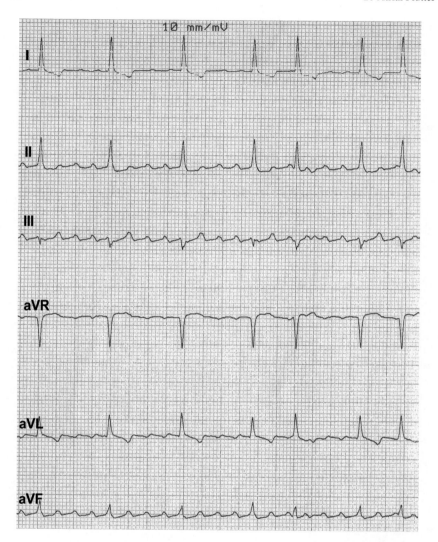

ECG 20.7 Electrocardiogram obtained from a 77-year-old woman with atrial flutter type 2 (positive flutter waves in III, aVF), with varying atrioventricular (AV) conduction (4:1 and 2:1 AV block, with superimposed Wenckebach phenomenon). Atrial rate 308 beats/min; ventricular rate approximately 77 and 154 beats/min, respectively

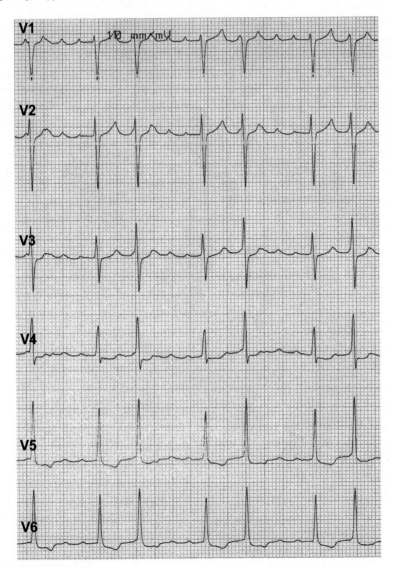

ECG 20.7 (continued)

atrial rate is also stable and may be faster, between 240 and 380 beats/min. The AV conduction shows the same variations as in the common type.

Because of the p wave-like flutter waves, uncommon atrial flutter is easily confounded with atrial tachycardia, which is even rarer than atrial flutter type 2. Because atrial tachycardia with incomplete AV block can result from digitalis intoxication, it is dangerous to give digitalis in such a case. Although the rate of atrial tachycardia rarely exceeds 210 beats/min, the differentiation between a fast atrial tachycardia and atrial flutter, especially of the uncommon type, is sometimes very difficult. Clinical findings, the patient's history, and the use of digitalis should be considered.

In common and uncommon atrial flutter, the electrophysiologic mechanism is a macroreentry within the right atrium. Flutter type 1 has a counterclockwise direction within the circuit and type 2 (inverse type 1) a clockwise direction.

Chapter 21
Atrial Fibrillation

After ventricular and atrial premature beats, atrial fibrillation (AF) is the most frequent arrhythmia. Hemodynamics and symptoms are related to the ventricular rate and the loss of atrial contraction. The most important complication of AF is cerebral stroke. Moreover, AF is an independent risk factor for death. Therapy and prevention of AF are complex.

Etiology and Prevalence

The most common etiology in chronic AF is fibrosis of the atrial myocardium in older patients. Other etiologies include all diseases with chronic overload of the left atrium, such as hypertensive heart disease, cardiomyopathies of any origin of the left ventricle, left-sided valvular diseases (especially mitral stenosis), and other conditions including hyperthyroidism, infections, and alcohol abuse. The prevalence of AF is 0.5%–0.8% at age 51–60 years and 9% at age 80–89 years.

Transient AF often occurs after open heart surgery (especially aortic and mitral valve surgery), in the acute stage of myocardial infarction, and in hyperthyreosis and alcohol abuse. AF rarely occurs in an otherwise normal heart. In this case, it is called "lone atrial fibrillation."

The only reliable diagnostic electrocardiogram (ECG) feature in AF is the absolutely irregular ventricular response, also called "absolute arrhythmia" (ECG 21.1). This compulsory sign is always detectable in a rhythm strip. Note the pitfalls: In tachyventricular AF, the rhythm may be almost regular (pseudo-regularization; ECG 21.2). In the very rare combination of AF with complete atrioventricular (AV) block and escape rhythm, the ventricular rhythm is regular. Of course, a regular ventricular rhythm is also seen in AF associated with ventricular pacing.

In most cases of AF, the f waves (fibrillatory waves) are clearly visible (for atrial flutter waves, the abbreviation "F waves" is used). The f waves are completely irregular in respect to rhythm and configuration and have a rate between 350 and 500 (up to 650) per minute. They are best detectable in leads V_1, III, and aVF. There

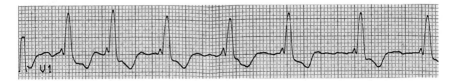

ECG 21.1 Electrocardiogram obtained from an 86-year-old woman. Lead V_1. Atrial fibrillation with the compulsory "absolute ventricular arrhythmia." The f waves are scarcely visible. Right bundle-branch block

ECG 21.2 Electrocardiogram obtained from a 75-year-old man. Leads V_2 and V_3. Pseudo-regularization of ventricular rhythm in tachycardic atrial fibrillation at a rate of approximately 180 beats/min. ST depression of 10 mm in V_2, probably the result of true ischemia and tachycardia

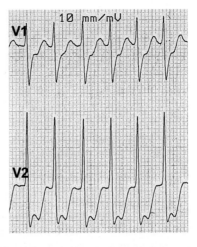

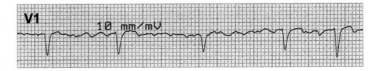

ECG 21.3 Electrocardiogram obtained from an 86-year-old woman. Lead V_1. Coarse f waves (fine waves at the beginning)

is a distinction between coarse f waves (ECG 21.3) and fine f waves (ECG 21.4), and occasionally, both are present in the same patient. However, there are some conditions for which f waves cannot be detected.

At very fast ventricular rates, the f waves are hidden within the QRS complex and the repolarization waves (ECG 21.2). The f waves may also be masked by a bundle-branch block, which leads to prolongation of the ventricular cycle (ECG 21.5). In the presence of fibrotic atria with only a small rest of myocardial fibers, the f waves are very small (ECG 21.6) or even lacking. In all these conditions, the correct diagnosis is made by the detection of absolute ventricular arrhythmia. In the presence of coarse f waves, the damage of the atrial muscle is generally less than in the presence of fine f waves and associated with a better short- and long-term success of direct current conversion.

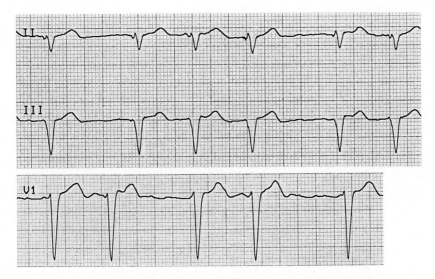

ECG 21.4 Electrocardiogram obtained from a 67-year-old man. Leads II, III, V₁. Fine f waves

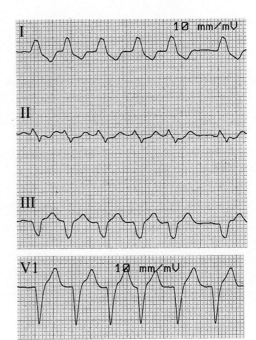

ECG 21.5 Electrocardiogram obtained from a 91-year-old woman. Leads I, II, III, V₁. No visible f waves in the presence of left bundle-branch block

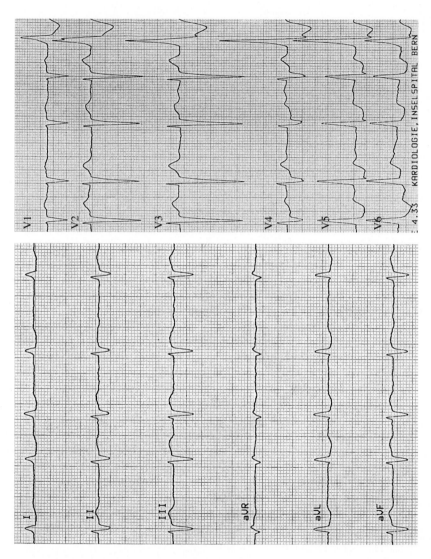

ECG 21.6 Electrocardiogram obtained from a 77-year-old man. Very small f waves in lead III (II, V$_1$). Left ventricular hypertrophy and ST depression in V$_5$/V$_6$ (V$_4$). The last beat is not an aberrant beat, but a ventricular premature beat (positive QRS deflection in all precordial leads)

Hemodynamics

Fortunately, not all atrial impulses (rate 350–650 beats/min) reach the ventricles. A large proportion of them is blocked in the AV node. The other impulses are conducted at random intervals to the ventricles, thus leading to the absolutely arrhythmic ventricular activity. A very fast, irregular ventricular activity has much clinical importance. Similar to very early ventricular premature beats, in every ventricular beat of AF with high instantaneous rate, the preceding diastole is shortened considerably, thus inhibiting a normal ventricular filling and consequently reducing the stroke volume, in extreme conditions to several milliliters. This means that not every QRS complex induces a ventricular contraction, sufficient for a palpable peripheric arterial pulse. The result is a "peripheric pulse deficit" that can reach >50% of the heart rate. The greater the peripheric pulse deficit, the smaller the cardiac output per minute.

Clinical Significance

AF is not necessarily a disease with symptoms and complications. Approximately half of the patients with AF have no restrictions in their daily life and never experience complications. The loss of the so-called atrial kick does not always cause symptoms. However, half of the patients have symptoms ranging from reduced work capacity, palpitations or even near syncope, to more or less severe complications, the most serious of which is cerebral stroke. The origin of embolism is thrombotic material within dilated atria, especially in the appendages. Whereas small pulmonary embolism is mostly asymptomatic, peripheric embolism often has serious consequences depending on the affected organs (cerebrum, intestine, limbs, very rarely coronary arteries). Moreover, AF may evoke or aggravate heart failure and it reduces survival, especially in patients with heart decompensation.

Symptoms generally result from an irregular ventricular response that is too slow or (more often) too fast. Syncope are rare and may occur with ventricular rates higher than 230 beats/min or during spontaneous conversion in sinus rhythm (ECG 21.7) caused by a longer atrial and ventricular standstill.

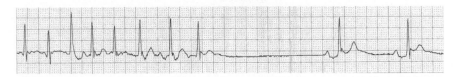

ECG 21.7 Electrocardiogram obtained from a 79-year-old man. Spontaneous conversion of atrial fibrillation. Ventricular pause before sinus rhythm 2.6 s

Aberrations in Atrial Fibrillation

Similar to any other case of supraventricular rhythm, AF may be conducted to the ventricles with every known aberration, such as bundle-branch block or fascicular block. However, two conditions, described below, are of special interest.

Ashman Beats

If a relatively long R-R interval is followed by a near QRS complex showing a bundle-branch block configuration, ventricular aberration is much more probable than a ventricular premature beat. This phenomenon is explained by the prolongation of the refractory period of the bundles by instantaneous bradycardia and was first described by Gouaux and Ashman as early as 1947. Ashman beats are most probable if the phenomenon can be observed several times on a longer rhythm strip. Right bundle-branch block aberration (ECG 21.8) is much more frequent than left bundle-branch block aberration, because the refractory period is longer in the right bundle than in the left. After an Ashman beat, a compensatory pause is lacking. This is in contrast to a ventricular premature beat that is usually followed by a compensatory pause. ECG 21.9 shows a repetitive aberration with left bundle-branch block imitating a ventricular tachycardia.

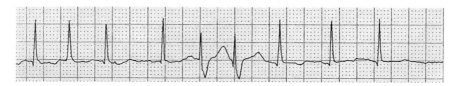

ECG 21.8 Lead II. Right bundle-branch block aberration for two beats, where the rate is faster than in the other beats. Aberration occurs after a relatively long R-R interval

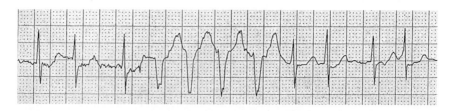

ECG 21.9 Lead V$_2$. Left bundle-branch block aberration for four beats, where the rhythm is slightly irregular and the rate relatively fast. Aberration occurs after a relatively long R-R interval. A ventricular tachycardia could be excluded

Atrial Fibrillation in Preexcitation
(Wolff-Parkinson-White Syndrome)

In both common "orthodromic" reentrant tachycardia and rare "antidromic" reentrant tachycardia, the accessory pathway ("AP") and the AV junction represent the circuit for conduction. In the first type, the AP is used for retrograde conduction and in the second type for antegrade conduction. The conduction of AF antegradely over an accessory pathway is rare but can represent the most extreme arrhythmia in patients with preexcitation. If the refractory time in antegrade conduction is very short, an abnormally high number of atrial impulses reaches the ventricles, with consequent excessive, fast ventricular activity and possible degeneration to ventricular fibrillation.

Often, a cautious analysis of the electrocardiogram allows the differentiation between a fast regular ventricular tachycardia or a supraventricular tachycardia with bundle-branch block on one hand, and tachyventricular AF with a preexcitation pattern (eventually with pseudo-regularization of the rhythm at a high rate) on the other hand. In the first conditions, delta waves are absent, but in the last case, delta waves are always present, usually best visible in the precordial leads (ECG 21.10). It is important to know that AF can occur in young patients and even in children with the Wolff-Parkinson-White syndrome, thus including the possibility of ventricular fibrillation. It is absolutely contraindicated to give digitalis or verapamil intravenously in AF combined with preexcitation. Both drugs slow conduction in the AV node and can enhance conduction antegradely in the accessory pathway. Death resulting from antegradely conducted AF (or atrial flutter with 1:1 conduction) along an accessory pathway, with consecutive ventricular fibrillation, is a rare but tragic event, especially in young persons. This is another reason why patients with Wolff-Parkinson-White syndrome should be investigated by invasive electrophysiology and ablation performed. (See also Chapter 24, The Wolff-Parkinson-White Syndrome.)

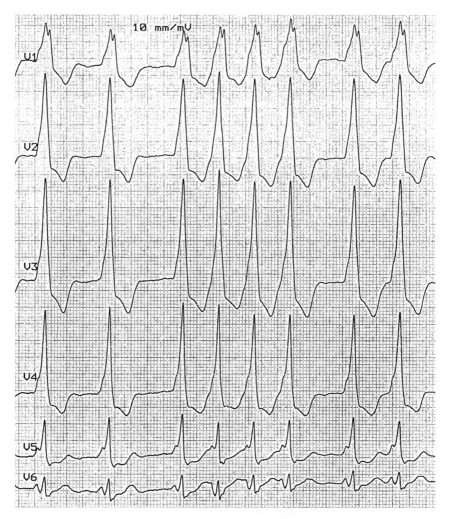

ECG 21.10 Electrocardiogram (ECG) obtained from a 72-year-old man. ECG (V_1 to V_6): atrial fibrillation in preexcitation (Wolff-Parkinson-White syndrome). The delta wave in V_6 imitates a p wave

Therapy of Atrial Fibrillation

The therapeutic approach to AF includes drugs, direct current conversion and ablation, or a combination of these. In most patients with AF, anticoagulation is necessary. The decision between rate control (with drugs) and electroconversion (rhythm control) has to be considered individually for each patient.

Chapter 22
Sick Sinus and Carotis Sinus Syndromes

Sick sinus syndrome is a disease of the sinus node, often with involvement of the surrounding conduction fibers and the atrioventricular (AV) node, and occurs, with exceptions, in middle- and older-aged patients. The likely predominant etiology is a degenerative process. Other etiologies include coronary heart disease (CHD), infectious diseases, and rare conditions. Clinically, the etiology remains unclear and is classified as "unknown." Carotis sinus syndrome is briefly discussed at the end of this chapter.

Characteristics of Sick Sinus Syndrome

Sick sinus syndrome represents a *collection* of electrocardiogram (ECG) signs, which include sinus bradycardia, sinus standstill/arrest, exit-block or sinuatrial (SA) block, and the bradycardia/tachycardia variant. Each of these is discussed below.

Sinus Bradycardia

The sinus rate for sinus bradycardia at rest is slower than 50 per minute. During exercise or under drug-induced sympathetic stimulation (with adrenaline or isoprenaline), the rate is slower than 90 per minute.

Sinus Standstill/Arrest

In sinus arrest, there is no impulse formation in the sinus node (ECG 22.1). In the ECG, sinus arrest can often be difficult to distinguish from SA block 2° or complete SA block. Longer episodes with absent p waves favor sinus arrest. Periodic absence of p waves are suspicious for SA block 2°.

M. Gertsch, *The ECG Manual: An Evidence-Based Approach*,
© Springer-Verlag London Limited 2009

Exit-Block or Sinuatrial Block

SA block is a conduction block within the sinus node or between the sinus node and its surrounding fibers, which normally conduct the sinus impulse to the atria and the AV node (ECG 22.2). Obviously, in cases with episodes of ventricular asystole, the AV junction is also involved, because an AV junction escape rhythm does not arise. As in AV block, SA block is subdivided in SA block 1°, two or three forms of SA block 2°, and complete SA block. Usually, only SA blocks 2° with 2:1 or 3:1 block are diagnosed in the routine ECG or in a Holter or monitor strip. Longer episodes of complete SA block cannot be distinguished from sinus arrest.

The Bradycardia/Tachycardia Variant

We find changes from bradycardic episodes (sinus arrest, SA block, sinus bradycardia) to episodes of tachycardia, including salvos of atrial premature beats, generally irregular atrial tachycardia, atrial flutter, atrial fibrillation and, rarely, AV nodal reentry tachycardias (ECG 22.3). Episodes of tachycardia generally occur as a reaction on bradycardia or are induced by atrial premature beats. Isolated atrial

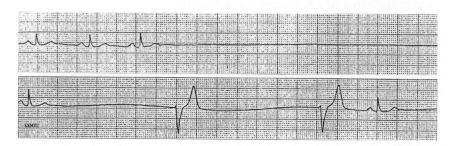

ECG 22.1 Continuous strip. Sinus standstill for approximately 7.5 s. After another sinusal beat, again sinus standstill. After probably two ventricular escape beats (instantaneous rate 21/min), one sinusal beat, then again sinus standstill

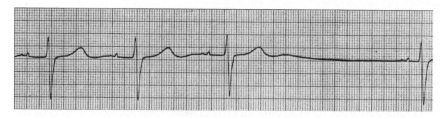

ECG 22.2 Paper speed 50 mm/s. Sinus rhythm (92 beats/min). Sinoatrial block 2:1. In this case, the p3–p4 interval exceeds the double preceding p-p intervals by 55 ms

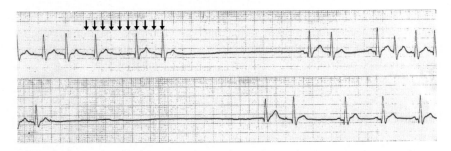

ECG 22.3 Brady-tachycardia variant. Continuous strip. Atrial flutter (irregular atrial action, rate about 300 beats/min; see arrows) with changing atrioventricular (AV) conduction. Stop of atrial flutter, sinus arrest during 3.24 s. Then sinusal beats and atrial premature beats (APBs). After a blocked APB, a second episode of atrial standstill lasting 5.2 s. Then one AV junction escape beat, one APB, sinus rhythm

fibrillation is in most cases a consequence of a hemodynamic overload or, in older people, of a fibrosis of the left atrium. Let us remember that the sinus node is situated in the right atrium. Atrial fibrillation in chronic and acute cor pulmonale is rare indeed. There are cases, however, in which atrial fibrillation represents a clinically important component of sick sinus syndrome. Often, several signs of sick sinus syndrome are detectable in the same patient (ECG 22.3).

The Atrioventricular Node and Bundle Branches in Sick Sinus Syndrome

In many cases, the AV node and the bundle branches are involved in the disease, with two consequences. First, the AV node often fails to act as an escape pacemaker during episodes of SA block or sinus standstill. Second, an additional AV block of all degrees and a bundle-branch block are present in approximately 16% of the sick sinus syndrome. The progression to complete AV block is 2.6% per year.

Clinical Significance

The diagnosis of sick sinus syndrome is made on the basis of the ECG abnormalities mentioned above. The clinical significance of sick sinus syndrome depends on the severity of symptoms such as palpitations, impaired work capacity, dizziness, presyncope, and syncope. Before therapy is performed, the correlation between the symptoms and the ECG abnormalities should be confirmed. Ambulatory ECG is the best diagnostic method, whereas electrophysiologic testing (determination of the sinus node recovery time and other parameters) is not as reliable as previously thought.

Sick sinus syndrome may be a very "capricious" disease, with either multiple attacks within a short time or long normal intervals. Thus, the result of ambulatory ECG may be false negative. In doubtful cases, a long-term ambulatory ECG (during 1 week) may be preferable.

Prognosis and Complications

Sick sinus syndrome is a chronic disease with a fairly rapid progression. Eventual syncopes are generally shorter than in the presence of complete AV block with asystolic episodes. The most important complication of the disease is a cerebral stroke, especially in cases associated with atrial fibrillation. A stroke is best prevented by oral anticoagulation. In contrast to chronic (especially infra-His) complete AV block, the chance for survival is much better in sick sinus syndrome. Survival in symptomatic sick sinus syndrome is impaired by stroke, heart failure, and complications of associated CHD.

Therapy

Drug therapy is problematic in patients with bradycardia and impossible in cases of the bradycardia/tachycardia variant. A pacemaker (dual chamber or AAI pacing in younger patients) is implanted in patients with symptoms and the ECG abnormalities. Pacing generally eliminates many symptoms, thus improving quality of life, but not significantly the survival. In the bradycardia-tachycardia variant, antiarrhythmic drugs must be added to avoid tachycardic episodes.

Differential Diagnosis of Sick Sinus Syndrome

Atrioventricular-Blocked Atrial Premature Beats

If a very early atrial premature beat is AV blocked and the ventricular pause measures approximately double the usual heart cycle *and* especially if the p wave is hidden in the previous T wave, an episode of SA block may be imitated (ECG 22.4).

Enhanced Vagal Tone

One or several episodes of cardiac asystole in patients within the first days after heart operations or during/shortly after other operations, only rarely correspond to a diseased sinus node. They are mainly caused by enhanced vagal tone and

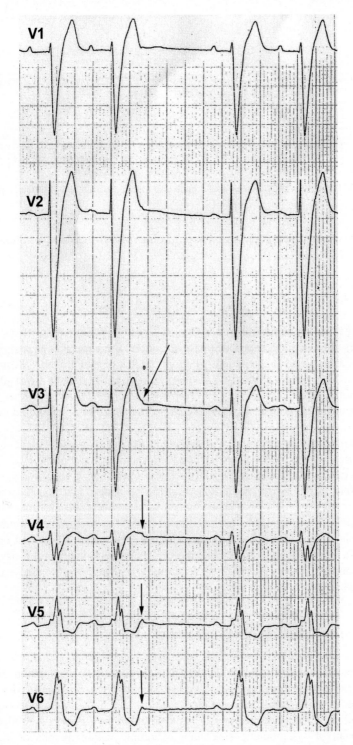

ECG 22.4 Sinus rhythm with atrioventricular (AV) block 1° and left bundle-branch block. AV blocked atrial premature beat, with the p wave detectable within/at the end of the T wave (arrow). The p-p interval is almost doubled (minus 55 ms)

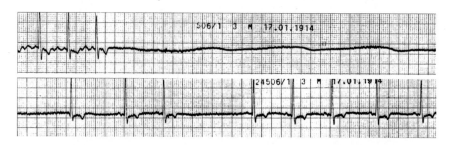

ECG 22.5 Short Story. Continuous strip. Sinus arrest with an atrial and ventricular pause of ≥9.7 s

disappear spontaneously. Also, temporary pacing is rarely needed (see Short Story and ECG 22.5).

Short Story/Case Report

A 68-year-old male patient had a sudden asystole, while sitting on a chair, 36 hours after an aortocoronary bypass operation. The nurse was alerted by the monitor and hurried to the patient who told her that he had probably slept for a moment. ECG stripe: sinus rhythm (mimicking atrial flutter) at a rate of 105 beats/min. Sudden sinus arrest, first escape beat after ≥9.7 s. After another short pause, sinus rhythm arose again (ECG 22.5). The patient was monitored during 48 hours, then two Holter ECGs were performed. No other asystole occurred and the patient was dismissed, without an electrophysiologic investigation or a pacemaker. He was well 4 years later and was then lost for control.

This case is extraordinary, not only because of the long pause. During vagal maneuvers (aspiration of tracheal secretion), the patient had no bradycardia. However, sitting calmly on a chair, sudden asystole occurred. The cause is not clear. An ECG artifact can be excluded by a discreet "warming up phenomenon" of the sinus node after the long pause and the occurrence of a second (short) pause. In view of the favorable outcome, the single episode of cardiac asystole corresponds to pseudo–sick sinus syndrome, despite the prolonged cardiac standstill.

"Laboratory" Sick Sinus Syndrome

In a few patients, without any symptoms related to sinus node dysfunction, electrophysiologic investigation reveals the typical electric characteristics of sick sinus syndrome, as prolonged sinus node recovery time and sinoatrial conduction time. Those patients should not receive a pacemaker, but clinical control is needed. The development of symptomatic sick sinus syndrome within months or years is possible.

Hypersensitive Carotid Sinus Syndrome

With the postmicturition syndrome, the "swallow syncope," and other conditions, the hypersensitive carotis sinus syndrome belongs to the great family of neurally mediated syncopal syndromes. The carotid sinus syndrome is found in older patients and is often associated with CHD. Two types are distinguished:

1. The *cardioinhibitory type* is defined as ventricular arrest of 3 s or more, occurring spontaneously or after carotid sinus massage. The ventricular pause is more often attributable to sinus arrest or to sinuatrial block (absence of QRS *and* p; ECG 22.6) than to sinus or atrial rhythm with complete AV block without AV junctional or ventricular escape rhythm (absence of QRS complexes and presence of p waves; ECG 22.7). Longer ventricular pauses lead to presyncope and syncope and are generally treated with a pacemaker, usually a double-chamber pacemaker. Asymptomatic patients, especially older patients with cardiac arrest of 3 s or more, provoked by carotid sinus massage, should not be treated with a pacemaker.

2. The *vasodepressor type* (vasodepressor carotid sinus hypersensitivity) is characterized by a decrease of systolic blood pressure of more than 30–50 mmHg, without rhythm disturbance, after carotid sinus massage. Symptomatic patients are treated with sodium-retaining drugs and elastic support hose, and in some cases with radiation or surgical denervation of the carotid sinus.

Cardioinhibitory and vasodepressive types can be combined. The mechanisms of carotid sinus syndrome include abnormal vagal function, baroreflex hypersensitivity, hyperresponsiveness to acetylcholine, among others. Rarely, hypersensitive carotid sinus syndrome and sick sinus syndrome are combined.

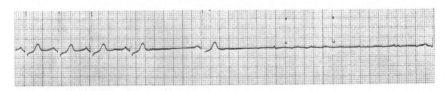

ECG 22.6 Carotid sinus massage leads to decrease of sinus rate and atrial standstill with ventricular asystole during 4.96 s. The small "spikes" during asystole correspond to artifacts and not to p waves. The last QRS is incomplete

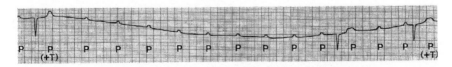

ECG 22.7 Carotid sinus massage induces complete atrioventricular (AV) block. After a ventricular asystole of 8.4 s, two AV junction escape beats arise, and shortly later, sinus rhythm (not shown)

Chapter 23
Atrioventricular Junctional Tachycardias

Some basic mechanisms of atrioventricular (AV) junctional tachycardias are presented in this chapter, along with discussion and demonstration of the enormous progress in electrophysiology and therapy of arrhythmias during the last two decades.

There are several types of AV junctional tachycardias, but most physicians are especially familiar with one type—the common *paroxysmal supraventricular tachycardia*, correctly referred to as *atrioventricular nodal reentrant tachycardia* (AVNRT). Note, however, that the supraventricular (reentry) tachycardia in **Wolff-Parkinson-White** (WPW) syndrome is called *atrioventricular reentry tachycardia*. AVNRT is based on the dual-pathway anatomy of the AV node. In a minority of humans, these two pathways are used functionally, in sinus rhythm as well as in AVNRT.

Conduction in Sinus Rhythm

The sinus impulse is conducted over the fast pathway beta, antegradely. At the same, the sinus impulse is also conducted antegradely over the slow pathway alpha. However, it is blocked, because the infra-AV nodal tissue is already activated by the sinus impulse over the fast pathway, and is therefore refractory (Figure 23.1).

Conduction in Atrioventricular Nodal Reentrant Tachycardia

In both pathways, retrograde conduction is also possible. Under certain circumstances, the two pathways are used as a reentry circuit, one pathway conducting antegradely, and the other retrogradely. The rate of this circuit movement is high, between 130 and 220/min. AVNRT is usually introduced by an atrial premature beat, often with AV block 1°.

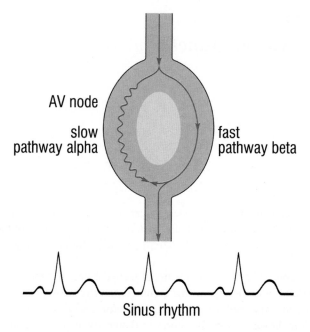

Figure 23.1 Dual atrioventricular (AV) pathway in sinus rhythm

There are two forms of AVNRT—common and rare. In both, the QRS complex is normal, and right bundle-branch block (RBBB) aberration is rare. The tachycardia is mainly absolutely regular. The rate is between 130 and 240 beats/min, often approximately 180 beats/min.

Common Form of Atrioventricular Nodal Reentrant Tachycardia

This tachycardia is paroxysmal and is responsible for >90% of AVNRTs, and for 50% of all regular supraventricular tachycardias. The slow pathway (alpha) is used for antegrade conduction, and the fast pathway (beta) for retrograde conduction. Therefore, the atria (retrogradely) and the ventricles (antegradely) are activated practically at the same time (Figure 23.2). Indeed, the p waves are completely hidden within the QRS complexes in approximately 70% of the cases (ECG 23.1) There is always an opposite P vector, compared with the normal sinus p vector, in the frontal plane: The p waves are negative in leads III, aVF, and often II, if they are not hidden within the QRS complex. In approximately 10% of the cases, the p waves are superimposed on the end of the QRS complex and are detectable as pseudo–s waves in the inferior leads aVF and III and/or as pseudo–r′ waves in lead

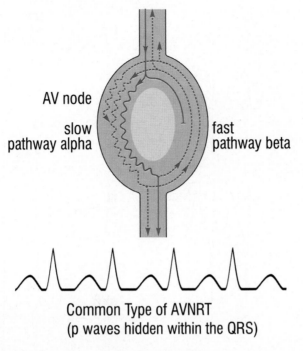

Figure 23.2 In the common type of atrioventricular nodal reentrant tachycardia (AVNRT), the slow pathway beta is used antegradely and the fast pathway alpha retrogradely

V_1, imitating incomplete RBBB (ECG 23.2). In approximately 20%, the p wave immediately follows the QRS complex and is visible within the ST segment or at the beginning of the T wave (ECG 23.3) The RP interval is always shorter than the PR interval (RP < PR).

The beginning (frequently induced by an atrial premature beat) and end of an episode of paroxysmal AVNRT is sudden ("light switch effect") and felt by most patients. Generally, the common type of AVNRT is encountered in younger individuals with an otherwise normal heart.

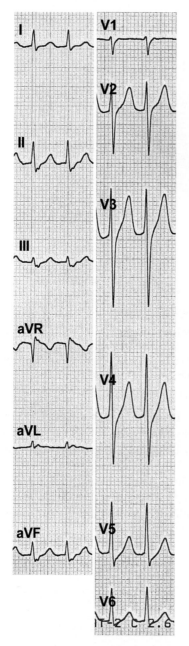

ECG 23.1 Electrocardiogram obtained from a 22-year-old man with an otherwise healthy heart. Atrioventricular nodal reentrant tachycardia, rate 158 beats/min. No detectable p waves

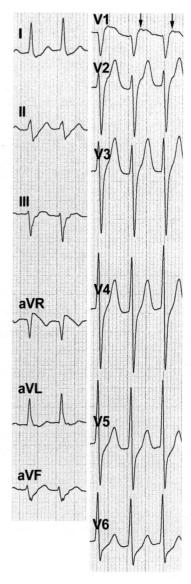

ECG 23.2 Electrocardiogram (ECG) obtained from a 28-year-old woman with an otherwise healthy heart. ECG: atrioventricular nodal reentrant tachycardia, rate 173 beats/min. The negative p waves are seen at the end of the QRS complex in II, aVF, III, formally broadening the S waves. Positive p wave after R in aVL. Moreover, p is seen as positive deflection in V_1, mimicking an r′ wave (see arrows) as in the pattern of incomplete right bundle-branch block

ECG 23.3 Electrocardiogram (ECG) obtained from a 44-year-old woman with hypertension. Moderate dilating cardiomyopathy. ECG: atrioventricular nodal reentrant tachycardia, rate 126 beats/min. The negative p waves are seen in the inferior leads and in all precordial leads, at the beginning of the T wave (the negative p waves in V_1/V_2 are unusual). Pathologic QRS configuration

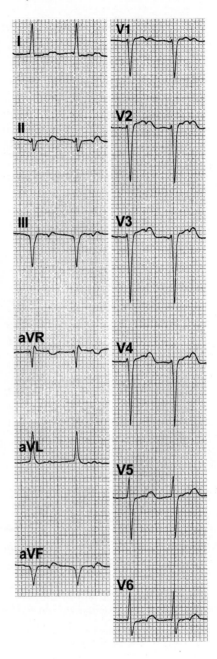

Rare Form of Atrioventricular Nodal Reentrant Tachycardia

This tachycardia may be *paroxysmal* or *incessant* (lasting many hours or days) and is responsible for only 5% of AVNRTs. The rare form of AVNRT occurs most often in heart disease. As the fast pathway (beta) is used antegradely and the slow pathway (alpha) retrogradely, the retrograde activation of the atria occurs later. Consequently, the negative p waves in the inferior leads aVF and III are often detectable, relatively late after the QRS complex (Figure 23.3). The RP interval is longer than the PR interval RP > PR) (ECG 23.4). The incessant form is often resistant to drugs and can lead to heart failure after days or months.

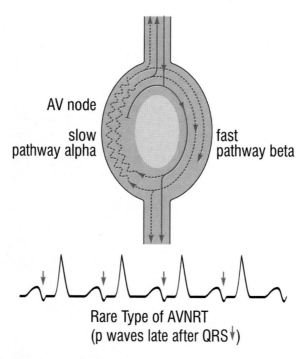

Figure 23.3   In the rare type of atrioventricular nodal reentrant tachycardia (AVNRT), the fast pathway alpha is used antegradely and the slow pathway beta retrogradely

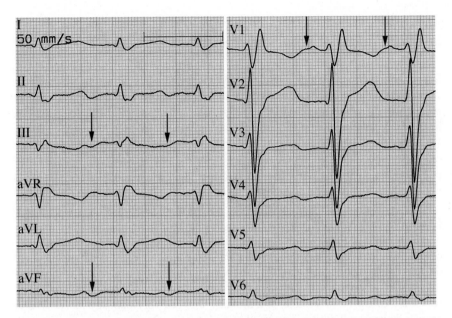

ECG 23.4 Electrocardiogram (ECG) obtained from a 32-year-old man with an otherwise normal heart. ECG: atrioventricular nodal reentrant tachycardia, rare type, rate 118 beats/min. The p waves (negative in III/aVF and positive in V_1) are seen *after* the T wave (RP > PR) (see arrow)

Differential Diagnosis

Theoretically, differential diagnosis includes all other forms of AV junction tachycardias along with atrial flutter and AV reentry tachycardia in the WPW syndrome. In practice, the other types of AV junction tachycardias (accelerated AV nodal rhythm, automatic junctional tachycardia, and permanent junctional reciprocating tachycardia) are so rare, especially in adults, that only atrial flutter and AV reentry tachycardia in the WPW syndrome are considered.

Atrial Flutter

Especially in flutter type 2 (with 1:1 or 1:2 AV conduction), the F waves are often not clearly detectable. Vagal maneuvers, especially carotis sinus massage, can enhance AV block and demask the flutter waves. In contrast, vagal maneuvers in AVNRT interrupt the tachycardia or have no effect. In sinus tachycardia with a high rate, carotid sinus massage slightly decreases the rate, for a short time.

Atrioventricular Reentry Tachycardia in Wolff-Parkinson-White Syndrome

Similar to the rare type of AVNRT, the atria in common WPW tachycardia are activated with some latency, because of the longer conduction from a ventricle to the atria. Thus, the p waves appear *after* the QRS, usually with RP < PR. As in the rare form of AVNRT, an RP > PR can also be present. In AV reentry tachycardia in WPW syndrome, only one "leg" of the dual AV conduction is used (mostly the fast one, antegradely); the other part of the reentry circuit is the accessory pathway, distant from the AV node (mostly with retrograde conduction). The majority of patients with WPW syndrome during sinus rhythm show a shortened PQ interval with the typical delta wave and more or less altered QRS and repolarization (see Chapter 24 on WPW syndrome).

The remarks thus far concerning the differential diagnosis based on the electrocardiogram, and especially on the behavior of the p wave, are theoretic to a certain degree. Every experienced cardiologist knows the obvious difficulties. In supraventricular tachycardias, especially at a high rate (and also without aberration), the p waves are often not detectable. Additionally, an accessory pathway in WPW syndrome can be occult during sinus rhythm. In fact, it is often impossible to differentiate among AVNRT, AV reentry tachycardia in WPW syndrome, and even atrial flutter (with 1:1 or 1:2 AV conduction). In those cases, an electrophysiologic investigation is mandatory for diagnosis and, of course, for therapy.

Aberration

In the case of an aberration (in general with an RBBB pattern), a ventricular tachycardia can be assumed, especially on the basis of a monitor lead. However, an aberration often occurs only during the first 3–10 beats (ECG 23.5). The different electrocardiogram signs in supraventricular tachycardias with RBBB and left bundle-branch block aberration ("SVTab") and ventricular tachycardia are discussed extensively in Chapter 26, "Ventricular Tachycardia."

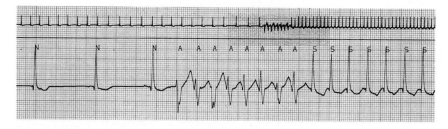

ECG 23.5 Electrocardiogram obtained from a 52-year-old man with coronary heart disease. Supraventricular tachycardia with aberration. The first eight beats (rate 180 beats/min) show right bundle-branch block aberration. After the rate decreases to 166 beats/min, the QRS complexes normalize. N, normal beats; A, beats with aberration; S, supraventricular beats

Symptoms and Clinical Significance of the Common Form of Atrioventricular Nodal Reentrant Tachycardia

Symptoms depend on the duration of the tachycardia. In general, the episodes last a few minutes, 30–60 min, or, exceptionally, many hours. Most patients experience tiresome palpitations and many feel the fast rate in the neck. This is caused by the contraction of the right atrium against a closed tricuspid valve that provokes visible pulsation of the external jugular veins ("a waves").

A high rate and/or a long duration of AVNRT may lead to dizziness, presyncope, and rarely syncope. Although the tachycardia is never directly life-threatening, it may be deleterious in situations such as swimming or mountain climbing, when tachycardia is associated with enhanced sympathetic tone.

Special Types of Atrioventricular Junctional Tachycardias

The other forms of AV junctional AV tachycardias, such as accelerated AV junctional rhythm, automatic junctional tachycardia, and the so-called permanent junctional reciprocating tachycardia, which is often classified as a variant of WPW syndrome, with an accessory pathway but without delta wave, are rare. These require individual electrophysiologic studies, and are not discussed here in detail.

Therapy of the Common Form of Atrioventricular Nodal Reentrant Tachycardia

Acute intravenous drug therapy is not always without danger. The most current drug in use is adenosine. However, some precautions should be taken; for instance, the dose should be reduced when using a central venous catheter. Verapamil has been widely used for many years, but can induce sudden asystole and even cardiogenic shock, and, in the presence of WPW syndrome, ventricular fibrillation. The vagal maneuvers such as Valsalva and carotid massage terminate the tachycardia in less than 40% of cases. Oftentimes, electroconversion is preferable.

The oral drug prophylaxis remains problematic. Today, the majority of patients with AVNRT with troublesome or severe symptoms are treated with catheter-induced radiofrequency ablation, which is successful in the first attempt nearly 95% of the time. Generally, the distal part of the slow pathway is interrupted. This curative therapy has considerably reduced urgent visits of physicians, particularly during the night.

Finally, the therapy for other types of AV junctional tachycardias depends on the mechanism of the arrhythmia.

Chapter 24
Wolff-Parkinson-White Syndrome

Preexcitation is based on an accessory conduction pathway between the atrium and ventricle. In the human embryo, there are three to four atrioventricular (AV) connections. Normally, all pathways, with exception of the AV node/His system, undergo hypoplasia or fibrosis and lose conduction function. However, in approximately 3 of every 1000 people, one so-called accessory pathway (AP) persists and can support antegrade and retrograde conduction. Generally, the electrocardiogram (ECG) in these individuals shows, constantly or more rarely intermittently, the typical pattern of preexcitation with a shortened PQ interval and a delta wave. Approximately 40% of the people with an AP experience tachycardias in which this pathway is used. The term *Wolff-Parkinson-White (WPW) syndrome* is used for patients with the preexcitation/WPW pattern associated with AP-related tachycardias.

Preexcitation Pattern

The preexcitation pattern or "WPW pattern" is characterized by the following:

1. A shortened PQ interval (PQ ≤0.12 s)
2. A typical delta wave
3. Deformation and prolongation of the whole QRS complex
4. Alterations of the repolarization

The preexcitation pattern corresponds to ventricular activation by atrial impulses, conducted along the AP (fusion beats, see below), formerly called Kent-bundle. Thus, the impulse "bypasses" the AV node and is conducted faster than normal to the ventricle (Figure 24.1). As a consequence of the preexcitation of the ventricles, the PQ interval is shortened and lasts ≤0.12 s. Moreover, the abnormal "eccentric" excitation of the ventricles leads to a deformation of the whole QRS complex and also to alteration of the repolarization. The initial part of the deformed QRS is called delta wave, according to its similarity to the Greek letter delta (ECG 24.1). The delta wave corresponds to the preexcited portion of one or both ventricles.

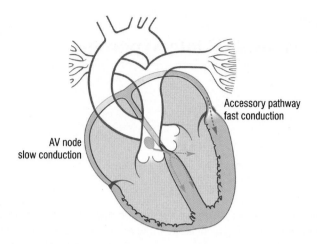

Figure 24.1 Preexcitation over the eccentric accessory pathway. AV, atrioventricular

Nomenclature

The traditional and simple previous nomenclature differentiates between types A and B. Type A shows an initially positive deflection in leads V_1/V_2 corresponding to early activation of the posterior left ventricle, and type B shows an initially negative deflection in V_1/V_2 corresponding to early activation of the anterior/superior right ventricle. Patterns with a negative delta wave in the left lateral leads V_5/V_6 have been called type C. The modern classification reflects more than a dozen different localizations of the APs (see Figure 24.2).

The polarity of the delta wave and the configuration of the whole QRS complex depends on the localization (site of origin and insertion) of the accessory pathway, which may be left-sided or right-sided, in the septal region, posterior or anterior/lateral. Consequently, both delta wave and the following part of the QRS can be positive, negative, or biphasic in some leads. In many cases, the localization of an AP can be predicted by the vectors of the delta waves and the QRS configuration. For detailed analysis, several algorithms have been developed.

The Electrocardiogram Patterns in Preexcitation

In WPW patients, three QRS patterns, discussed below, can be seen in the sinus rhythm.

1. Most preexcitation patterns represent fusion beats. The ventricles are activated at the same time along the AP and the AV node. The QRS configuration depends on the grade of activation along the AP and the AV node, respectively. The more

ECG 24.1 Electrocardiogram obtained from a 60-year-old woman. Sinus rhythm, typical preexcitation with shortened PQ interval (0.11 s) and positive delta wave, best seen in V_2 to V_6. (Note: In aVF and III, the delta waves are negative, because of projections.) QRS duration 160 ms. Alteration of repolarization

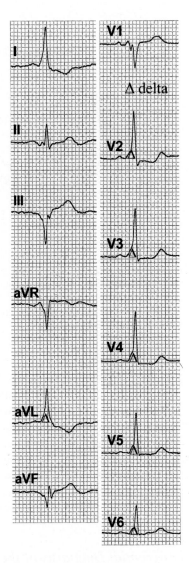

ventricular tissue is activated along the AP, the more similar the QRS complex is to the classical preexcitation pattern (ECG 24.1). The more ventricular tissue is activated along the AV node, the more similar the QRS complex is to a normal configuration (ECG 24.2). Thus, in the case of 90% ventricular activation along the AV node, the preexcitation pattern might be difficult to detect. We could find an only modestly reduced PQ interval, only an "abortive" delta wave, and a minor alteration of the whole QRS complex and the repolarization (ECG 24.2). Also, the same patient might show different grades of preexcitation in his or her ECGs, with more or less typical preexcitation.

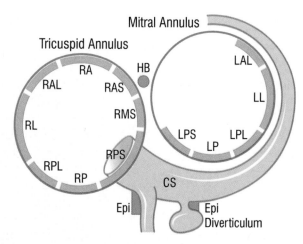

Figure 24.2 Diagram of accessory pathway location. Schematic cross-section of the ventricles at the level of the atrioventricular valve rings in left anterior oblique projection. CS, coronary sinus; HB, His bundle; RAS, right anteroseptal; RMS, right midseptal; RPS, right posteroseptal; RP, right posterior; RPL, right posterolateral; RL, right lateral; RAL, right anterolateral; RA, right anterior; LAL, left anterolateral; LL, left lateral; LPL, left posterolateral; LP, left posterior; LPS, left posteroseptal; Epi, epicardial

2. In rare cases, there might be *full* preexcitation. The ventricles are activated exclusively along the AP. The ECG pattern is very typical (ECG 24.3).
3. In approximately 30% of WPW patients, the AP conducts only retrogradely. The term "concealed AP" is used. In theses cases, the PQ interval and the QRS complex are normal and the diagnosis cannot be made on the basis of an ECG, but only by electrophysiologic studies (e.g., in patients with paroxysmal supraventricular tachycardias). In contrast to patients with manifest WPW pattern *and* syndrome where atrial fibrillation (AF) is found in up to 32% (lifetime prevalence), these patients have concomitant AF in only about 3%.

Differential Diagnosis of the Wolff-Parkinson-White Pattern

Myocardial Infarction

In more than 50% of cases, the WPW pattern leads to pathologic Q waves that could be confounded with a previous myocardial infarction (MI). However, the shortened PQ interval and the delta wave suggest the true diagnosis. Moreover, the T waves are discordant positive in the leads with pathologic Q waves and not concordant negative as usual in previous MI.

A complete negative QRS complex (QS) with a negative delta wave in leads III and aVF may imitate the pattern of a previous inferior MI (ECG 24.4). Tall R waves in V_1 to V_3 suggest posterior MI (ECG 24.5), whereas the combination of such

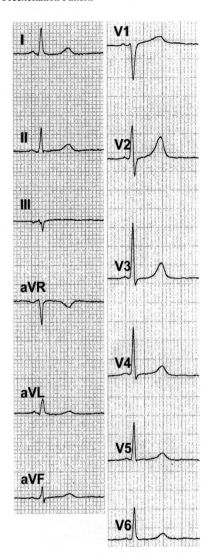

ECG 24.2 Electrocardiogram (ECG) obtained from a 56-year-old woman. Sinus rhythm, PQ interval approximately 0.11 s. Questionable "abortive" delta waves in V_2/V_3. Similar patterns are seen as normal variants (pseudo–delta waves, because of projection of a normal QRS; see Chapter 3), albeit with a normal PQ

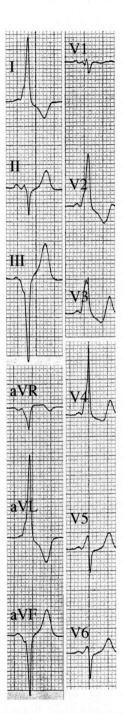

ECG 24.3 Electrocardiogram obtained from a 6-year-old girl. "Full" preexcitation, with enormous deformation of QRS and of repolarization

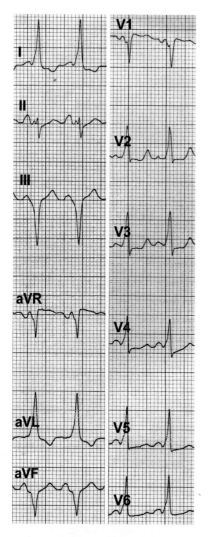

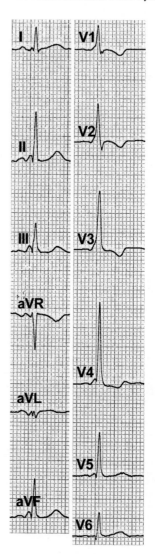

ECG 24.4 Electrocardiogram obtained from a 29-year-old woman. Sinus tachycardia, PQ 0.10 s, delta waves. QS in III/aVF formally imitates inferior myocardial infarction. Note: The T wave is positive

ECG 24.5 Electrocardiogram obtained from a 24-year-old man. Sinus rhythm, typical preexcitation. Tall R waves in V_1 to V_3 imitate posterior myocardial infarction. Note biphasic delta waves in several leads

patterns imitates inferoposterior MI (ECG 24.6). Also, (postero-)lateral MI can be mimicked (ECG 24.7). In patients with preexcitation, the presence of a previous infarction is not recognizable in general. The pattern of acute MI can occasionally be detected on the basis of striking ST elevations.

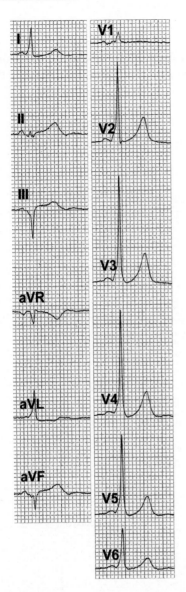

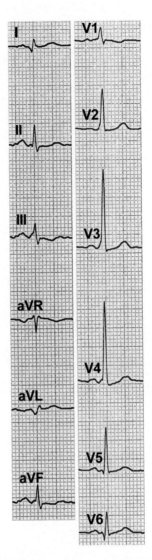

ECG 24.6 Electrocardiogram obtained from a 63-year-old man. Sinus rhythm, typical preexcitation. QS in III/aVF and tall R waves in V_1 to V_3 might be falsely interpreted as inferoposterior myocardial infarction, and the giant R waves in V_2 to V_5 as concentric left ventricular hypertrophy

ECG 24.7 Electrocardiogram obtained from a 56-year-old man. Sinus rhythm, typical preexcitation. Significant Q waves in I/aVL (and V_6) and tall R waves in V_1 to V_3 imitate posterolateral myocardial infarction

Left Ventricular Hypertrophy

Often, preexcitation enhances the R wave voltage (especially in the precordial leads), thus suggesting left ventricular hypertrophy (ECG 24.8). In these cases, the strain pattern with asymmetric negative T waves might also be observed.

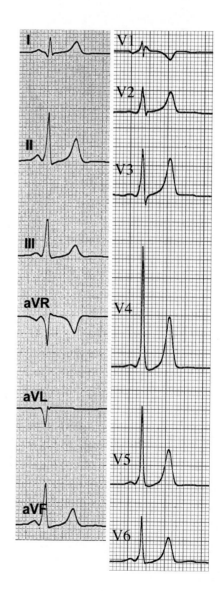

ECG 24.8 Electrocardiogram obtained from a 57-year-old man. Typical preexcitation. Tall R wave in V$_4$ might suggest left ventricular hypertrophy

Pseudo–Delta Wave

Occasionally a pseudo–delta wave is present in leads V_2 and V_3, and/or in the inferior leads, because of projection. In these cases, the PQ interval and the QRS complex are normal (see also Chapter 3 regarding the normal ECG).

Tachycardias in the Wolff-Parkinson-White Syndrome

Reentry Tachycardias

The typical tachycardias in the WPW syndrome are based on a *macro*-reentry using the AP and the AV node. Two types are distinguished:

1. In >90% of cases, the impulse is conducted retrogradely along the AP and antegradely along the AV node (Figure 24.3a). This type is called orthodromic

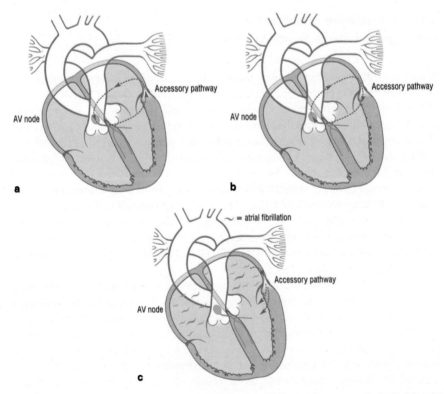

Figure 24.3 Diagram of accessory pathway location. **a.** Orthodromic tachycardia **b.** Antidromic tachycardia **c.** Tachycardia in atrial fibrillation (short refractory period of the accessory pathway). AV, atrioventricular

reentry tachycardia. Consequently, the QRS is normal (in absence of an additional bundle-branch block) and a delta wave is always missed (ECG 24.9). The distinction from AV nodal reentrant tachycardia is often not possible without electrophysiologic investigation. A negative p wave in lead V_1, shortening of the R-R interval in the case of disappearing ipsilateral bundle-branch block, and an RP > PR interval, favor WPW syndrome.

2. In <10% of the cases, the AP is used antegradely and the AV node retrogradely. This type is called antidromic reentry tachycardia (Figure 24.3b). In these rare cases, the QRS complex corresponds to the typical WPW pattern, a delta wave included (ECG 24.10).

In both antidromic and orthodromic tachycardia, the rhythm is regular and the rate is between 140 and 240 beats/min (ECG 24.9) and occasionally reaches nearly 250 beats/min (ECG 24.11) or even 300 beats/min. At rates up to 220 beats/min, negative p waves may be detected in the inferior leads III and aVF, because of retrograde atrial activation, with RP > PR.

Atrial Fibrillation and Flutter in Wolff-Parkinson-White Syndrome

In patients with especially manifest preexcitation in the ECG (in sinus rhythm), AF is common and is even described in children. Tachycardias caused by AF and atrial flutter do not represent a reentry tachycardia (see below). However, these arrhythmias are clinically very important, because of possible degeneration into ventricular fibrillation, in the case of a very short (antegrade) refractory period of the AP.

Only the AP is used for conduction, antegradely, and there is no manifest retrograde conduction over the AV junction (Figure 24.3c). Therefore, delta waves and wide, deformed QRS are present during tachycardia. In AF, the ventricular rhythm is absolutely irregular (ECG 24.12a). The patient represented in ECG 24.12b was registered during infusion with procainamide. Because of the slowing rate, some stimuli are conducted over the AV node, others over the AP, and some are fusion beats. After conversion to sinus rhythm (ECG 24.12c), the preexcitation pattern is scarcely detectable at first glance.

AF with preexcitation must be distinguished from monomorphic ventricular tachycardia, for which the rhythm is regular. Rarely, in ventricular tachycardia, a slow upstroke of wide QRS can imitate a delta wave. The ventricular rate in AF or atrial flutter depends on antegrade conduction properties of the AP. If the refractory period is very short, the ventricular rate could reach up to 300 beats/min in AF and in atrial flutter with 1:1 conduction. At these extreme rates, degeneration into ventricular fibrillation could occur as a result of severely impaired coronary perfusion.

ECG 24.9 Electrocardiogram obtained from a 48-year-old man. Wolff-Parkinson-White syndrome. Orthodromic tachycardia, rate 185 beats/ min. The QRS are normal (no delta wave, because the "accessory pathway" is used retrogradely). No visible p waves. Incomplete right bundle-branch block

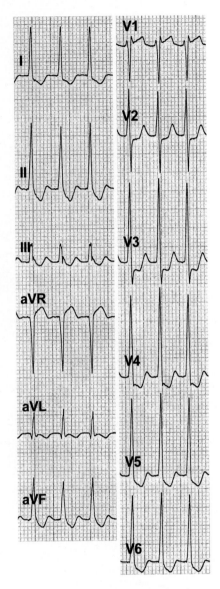

Although only a minority of patients with WPW tachycardia present a very fast antegrade conduction over the AP, allowing an extremely rapid ventricular response, the typical ECG pattern must be recognized, for therapeutic reasons as well.

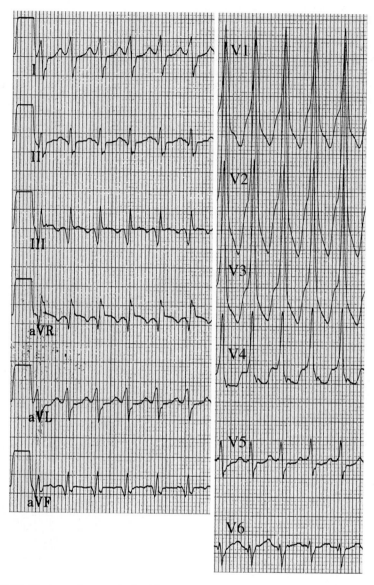

ECG 24.10 Electrocardiogram obtained from a 75-year-old woman. Antidromic atrioventricular reentry tachycardia, rate 185 beats/min. The QRS complexes are fully preexcited and indicate the location of the accessory pathway (left lateral)

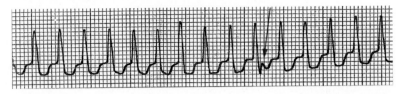

ECG 24.11 Electrocardiogram obtained from a 40-year-old man. Wolff-Parkinson-White syndrome. Rhythm strip. Orthodromic tachycardia, rate 238 beats/min. Arrow: artifact

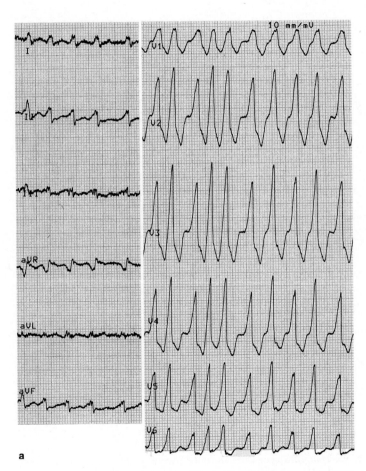

ECG 24.12 Electrocardiogram (ECG) obtained from a 45-year-old woman. The patient came to the emergency unit because of a presyncope during palpitations. **a.** ECG: atrial fibrillation with absolute ventricular arrhythmia and wide QRS; maximal instantaneous rate 268 beats/min. No clear delta waves, however relative slow R upstroke in many complexes (see leads V_2 to V_6). A Wolff-Parkinson-White syndrome was not known but diagnosed on the basis of this ECG

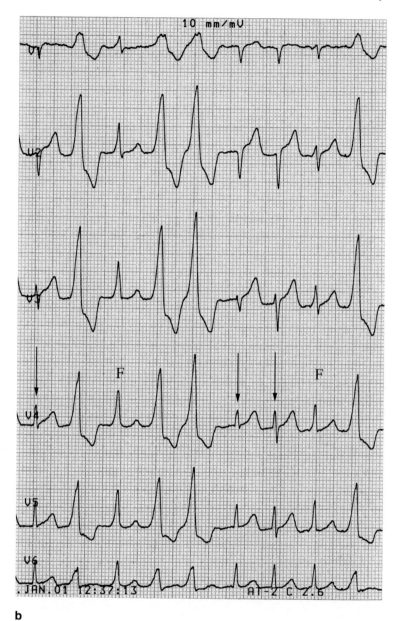

b

ECG 24.12 (continued) **b.** ECG (V_1 to V_6) during infusion of procainamide. Slower rate, persisting arrhythmia. Four QRS complexes show the pattern of "full preexcitation," three beats are conducted over the AV node (arrow), two beats are fusion beats (F).

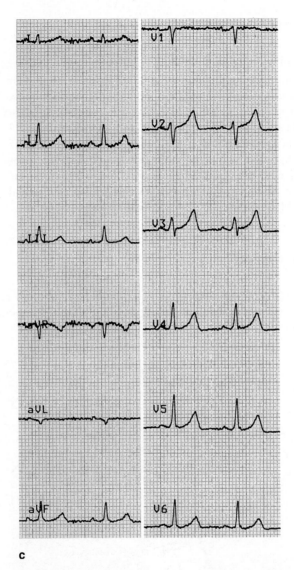

c

ECG 24.12 (continued) **c.** ECG after conversion to sinus rhythm (SR) with procainamide. Although the patient had a potentially life-threatening arrhythmia, her ECG in SR shows only a "minor" pattern of preexcitation, not initially recognizable

Symptoms and Therapy

The majority of patients with the WPW syndrome show symptoms that depend on duration and especially on the rate of tachycardia. The symptoms include palpitations, dizziness, presyncope, and syncope. Symptomatic patients should undergo electrophysiologic evaluation and catheter ablation (approximately 95% successful). In patients refusing ablation, one has to resort prophylactically to active drugs such as flecainide, propafenone, and beta-blockers. For interruption of a WPW tachycardia, we prefer an electroconversion or procainamide. Digitalis and verapamil are contraindicated in patients with WPW syndrome, especially in the presence of AF. These drugs impair AV conduction and can enhance conduction over the AP by shortening the antegrade refractory time.

Other Bypass Tracts

Two different Mahaim fibers, the James fiber, and other tracts may be responsible for extremely rare tachycardias (Figure 24.4). For more information about the WPW syndrome, see specific literature.

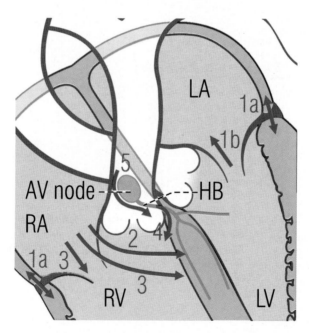

Figure 24.4 Different varieties of conducting bypass tracts. Arrows indicate direction of propagation; 4 and 5, if they exist, are extraordinarily rare. 1a, Kent bundle; 1b, concealed accessory pathway (Kent); 2, atriofascicular fiber (Mahaim); 3, atrioventricular fiber (Mahaim, "accessory AV node"); 4, true Mahaim fiber; 5, James fiber; AV, atrioventricular; RA, right atrium; LA, left atrium; RV, right ventricle; LV, left ventricle; HB, His bundle

Therapeutic Pitfalls

Drugs, especially digitalis or verapamil, not only slow antegrade conduction along the AV node but can accelerate conduction along the AP, thus inducing an extremely high ventricular rate and consecutive degeneration into ventricular fibrillation. Many case reports have been published about an adverse outcome of trials of tachycardia conversion with these drugs. Digitalis and verapamil (especially intravenously administered) are absolutely contraindicated in patients with WPW syndrome.

This is also true for a patient in whom a typical AV reentry tachycardia in known WPW syndrome (or in WPW tachycardia misdiagnosed as atrioventricular nodal reentrant tachycardia) has been interrupted successfully in the past, e.g., with verapamil. This patient could suddenly present AF or atrial flutter that is difficult to diagnose in the ECG. Let us remember that atrial flutter and especially AF is more frequent in patients with WPW than in those without WPW (lifetime prevalence up to 32%). AF can occur during a common regular WPW tachycardia, by enhanced sympathetic tone, stress to the left atrium, and impaired coronary flow.

Special Bypass Tracts

Whereas Mahaim Tachycardia represents an extremely rare tachycardia that is connected with a special bundle and combined with left bundle-branch block morphology, the so-called *Lown-Ganong-Levine syndrome* (normal or slightly shortened PQ interval with paroxysmal supraventricular tachycardias) has found several electrophysiologic explanations and its existence was even doubted by several authors.

Chapter 25
Ventricular Premature Beats

Ventricular premature beats (VPBs) represent the most frequent arrhythmia by far. VPBs are found in approximately 60% of healthy people in an ambulatory electrocardiogram (Holter ECG). In these cases, the VPBs are generally single and monomorphic; the number does not exceed 100 (or perhaps as high as 200) per hour. In heart diseases, VPBs occur at a rate of 80%–90%, isolated or in salvos. VPBs may be monomorphic or polymorphic in these cases.

Definition and Nomenclature

VPBs are characterized by a *premature broad QRS complex* (generally QRS duration ≥120 ms) without a preceding p wave. A p wave occurring immediately before a broad QRS is not conducted unless preexcitation is present. Small QRS with only slightly altered configuration are encountered in VPBs arising in the interventricular septum.

In *bigeminy* (ECG 25.1), every normal beat is followed by a premature beat (1:1 extrasystole). In *trigeminy*, every normal beat is followed by two premature beats (ECG 25.2). In *quadrigeminy*, every normal beat is followed by three premature beats. In *2:1 extrasystole*, a premature beat occurs after two normal beats (ECG 25.3), and in *3:1 extrasystole*, a premature beat occurs after three normal beats (ECG 25.4). In several textbooks, the differences among the sequences of normal and premature beats are not defined. However, hemodynamics are more compromised (ECG 25.5) and the heart is generally sicker in trigeminy/quadrigeminy than in 2:1/3:1 extrasystole.

Two consecutive VPBs are called a *couplet*, three consecutive VPBs are called a *triplet*. Three or more consecutive VPBs are called *ventricular tachycardia*. With up to approximately four consecutive VPBs the expression *salvos* is also used. VPBs arise in one of the ventricles and occasionally in the interventricular septum and can show a normal QRS duration.

M. Gertsch, *The ECG Manual: An Evidence-Based Approach*,
© Springer-Verlag London Limited 2009

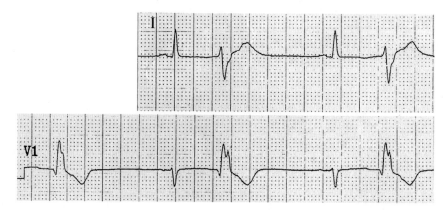

ECG 25.1 Ventricular premature beats in bigeminy. Leads I and V$_1$. Right bundle-branch block–like pattern with qR in V$_1$

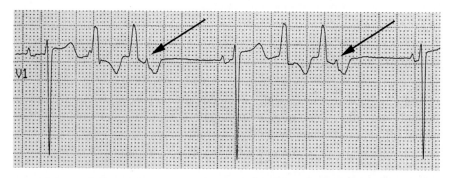

ECG 25.2 Ventricular premature beats in trigeminy. Lead V$_1$. Right bundle-branch block–like pattern with R in V$_1$, QS complex in V$_6$ (not shown). Atrioventricular dissociation detectable in V$_1$ (arrow)

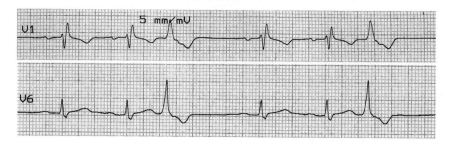

ECG 25.3 Leads V$_1$/V$_6$. Ventricular 2:1 extrasystole. Purely positive QRS in the precordial leads. In sinus rhythm, there is atrioventricular block 1° and incomplete right bundle-branch block

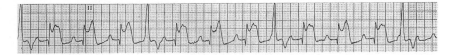

ECG 25.4 Electrocardiogram obtained from a 44-year-old man with acute anterior myocardial infarction. Lead II, continuous strip: ventricular 3:1 extrasystole. Note alternating repolarization (as a sign of ischemia), interrupted by ventricular premature beats. Other strips showed bigeminy. Thus, concealed bigeminy is probably present

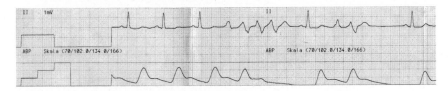

ECG 25.5 Continuous strip. Upper strip: rhythm. Lower strip: blood pressure. In this case, only the first ventricular premature beat leads to normal left ventricular contraction. The subsequent ventricular premature beat(s) remain without hemodynamic response

Coupling Interval

In general, the coupling intervals of VPBs show no or only modest differences (up to approximately 60 ms). Changing coupling intervals are observed in polytopic VPBs. If "monomorphic" VPBs show considerably different coupling intervals, ventricular parasystole is probable and can be confirmed by detecting an independent regular slower ventricular rhythm, with the help of a pair of dividers.

Compensatory Pause

In VPBs, all ventricular impulses are conducted retrogradely to the atria, at least partially. Approximately 50% are discharging the sinus node. If the impulse does not interfere with the sinus rhythm, the next sinusal impulse is delivered after a normal interval. The cycle is referred to as fully compensatory. However, a slightly earlier onset of the sinusal beat is common (not fully compensatory cycle).

Morphology and Origin

Monomorphic VPBs originate from the same focus and are called *unifocal* (ECG 25.6). *Polymorphic VPBs* might be unifocal with varying ventricular activation (the coupling interval is equal), or multifocal (varying coupling intervals, shown in ECG 25.7).

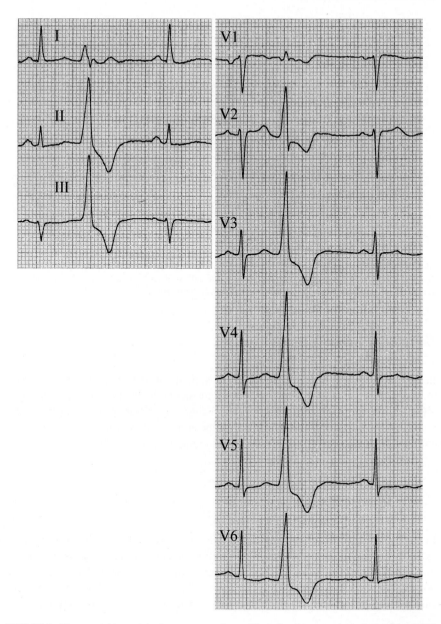

ECG 25.6 Monomorphic ventricular premature beats. Note the almost exclusively positive QRS in precordial leads

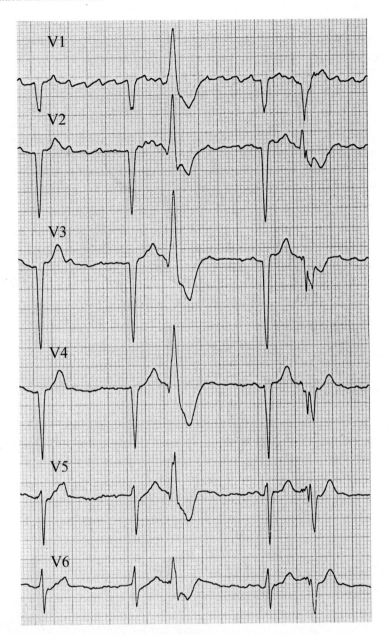

ECG 25.7 Electrocardiogram (ECG) obtained from a 76-year-old man. ECG: Polymorphic ventricular premature beats. Atrial fibrillation

It is often stated that VPBs with a right bundle-branch block (RBBB)-like pattern originate in the left ventricle and VPBs with a left bundle-branch block (LBBB)-like pattern in the right ventricle. This concept contradicts the reflection that follows. Because the diseases of the left ventricle are much more frequent than those of the right ventricle overall, the prevalence of VPBs with a RBBB-like pattern should exceed by far that of VPBs with a LBBB-like pattern. Because this is not true, more complex mechanisms (such as the site of the breakthrough phenomenon of the electric impulse) are responsible for the QRS configuration. However, the concept mentioned previously is quite reliable in some conditions. In arrhythmogenic right ventricular dysplasia, VPBs or a ventricular tachycardia (VT) with an LBBB-like pattern is generally found, and for VPBs or a VT originating in the right ventricular outflow tract, an LBBB-like pattern with a vertical frontal QRS axis is typical.

A superior QRS axis generally reflects an origin near the left posterior fascicle or at the base of one ventricle, and a vertical QRS axis reflects an origin near the left anterior fascicle or at the right ventricular outflow tract. In the rare VPBs originating in the interventricular septum and conducted near normally over the right bundle branch and the left fascicles, the QRS complex is narrow.

Special Types of Ventricular Premature Beats

R on T Phenomenon

A VPB, falling on the T wave early (earlier than approximately 90% or 85% of the preceding QT interval), is called *R on T*. Such a VPB can induce a VT (ECG 25.8) or even ventricular fibrillation, especially in the ischemic myocardium.

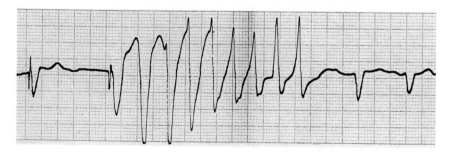

ECG 25.8 Electrocardiogram obtained from an 86-year-old man with a pacemaker. R on T. Rhythm strip. A ventricular premature beat falling on the T wave immediately after the apex induces a short ventricular tachycardia of the type torsades de pointes

Short Story/Case Report

On April 12, 2000, a 78-year-old male patient had an acute anteroseptal infarction. Because of persisting angina despite adequate drug therapy, he was transferred from a regional hospital to the university clinic 10 days later. Coronary angiography revealed a severe three-vessel disease with proximal stenosis; the left ventricular ejection fraction was moderately decreased (50%). A triple aortocoronary bypass operation was performed 1 day later. The postoperative course was uneventful; the monitored ECG showed only some banal VPBs. The patient was transferred to the general department. A 12-lead ECG on day 5 after operation showed numerous monomorphic VPBs with an extremely short coupling interval, an excessive R on T phenomenon (ECG 25.9a). The patient was

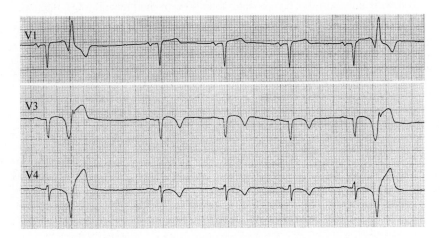

a

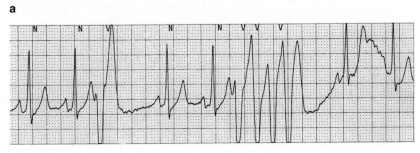

b

ECG 25.9 Electrocardiograms (ECGs) obtained from a 78-year-old man, described in the Short Story. **a.** R on T phenomenon. ECG (leads V_1, V_3, and V_4): sinus rhythm, 63 beats/min. Single ventricular premature beats (VPBs) falling into, or even slightly before, the apex of the T wave. **b.** Monitor strip: sinus rhythm, 93 beats/min. VPBs falling distinctly after the T apex. The third VPB induces a short ventricular tachycardia (VT), with "true R on T phenomenon," at a maximal instantaneous rate of about 280 beats/min. However, during fast VT, this phenomenon is common, also without being a precursor of ventricular fibrillation

ECG monitored and amiodarone was given perorally. During the next night, shortly after some fast ventricular runs (ECG 25.9b), the patient developed two episodes of ventricular fibrillation and had to be reanimated electromechanically. Amiodarone was given intravenously and perorally. The re-coro revealed open bypasses but a new stenosis (plaque rupture?) of the circumflexa artery, distally to the graft. Percutaneous coronary transluminal angioplasty was performed. Thereafter, relevant arrhythmias and R on T phenomenons on the ECG monitor and in a Holter ECG had disappeared. Five days later, the patient was dismissed home, with amiodarone 200 mg/day. Four years later, he was well (taking amiodarone, 100 mg/day).

A "visual" extreme R on T phenomenon is also seen in atrial fibrillation at a high instantaneous rate (>220 beats/min). In these cases, we have never observed ventricular fibrillation, except in Wolff-Parkinson-White syndrome.

If a VPB falls into the T wave later than 90% of the preceding QT interval, the term *R on T* is fulfilled. However, in this case, the VPB falls into the "supernormal period" and *not* into the "potential vulnerable period" of repolarization. Those R on T phenomenons are always harmless and are also seen in healthy individuals.

Interponated Ventricular Premature Beats

Rarely, a VPB does not interfere with the following normal beat. We miss a postextrasystolic pause (ECG 25.10). Interponated (or interpolated) VPBs do not have any special significance.

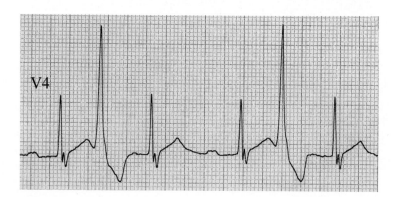

ECG 25.10 Electrocardiogram (ECG) obtained from a 45-year-old man. Uncomplicated atrioventricular (AV) channel. ECG, lead V_4 (4 days after surgical correction): Interponated ventricular premature beat (VPB) in 2:1 sequence. Purely positive QRS in all precordial leads (not shown). No postextrasystolic pause. AV block 1° and right bundle-branch block. The PQ time (0.32 s) is equal before and after VPB. Note that in interponated VPBs, the PQ interval is generally prolonged in the postextrasystolic beat

Fusion Beat

Simultaneous activation of the ventricles by a ventricular and supraventricular stimulus leads to a fusion beat. The QRS duration is between that of the supraventricular beat and that of the VPB. The morphology generally shows signs of the supraventricular and ventricular QRS complex, similarly to a child that shows characteristics of the mother *and* the father. Fusion is an important phenomenon, which is seen in late (phase 4) VPBs, in preexcitation and as a diagnostic sign in VT (here also called *Dressler beats*), accelerated idioventricular rhythm, and parasystole.

Concealed Bigeminy

In long rhythm strips with bigeminy, periods without bigeminy might be observed. If the number of the supraventricular (most sinusal) beats between the VPBs is odd, concealed bigeminy can be assumed (ECG 25.11). After every second sinusal beat, a premature beat is generated but not conducted and therefore invisible in the ECG. Concealed bigeminy does not impair the hemodynamics, as bigeminy often does, but represents an additional disturbance of conduction. It can be a result of drug treatment of bigeminy.

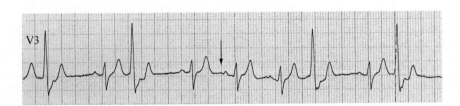

ECG 25.11 Concealed bigeminy (lead V_3). Ventricular premature beats (VPBs) in bigeminy, except during three consecutive sinusal beats. A blocked VPB (arrow) is probable. In this case, the coupling interval of the VPBs is not constant

Differential Diagnosis of Ventricular Premature Beats

VPBs have to be distinguished from supraventricular premature beats with a broad QRS. In the latter, broad QRS are caused by aberrant ventricular conduction, generally RBBB or LBBB aberration. In many cases, a preceding p wave can be identified, with a normal or prolonged PR interval. Often, the p waves are hidden within the T wave and can be detected by a deformation of the T wave, which is either pointed or "camel-like." Atrioventricular nodal premature beats with aberration are very rare. In this case, p waves are hidden within the QRS complex, because of retrograde activation of the atrias. Differentiation from VPBs might be possible by respective QRS morphology in the precordial leads. In VPBs, the bundle block pattern is atypical (see Chapter 26).

Therapy

Since the publication by Velebit et al. (Circulation, 1982) and especially since the CAST Study (N Engl J Med, 1989), the medical world has recognized that "cosmetic treatment" of VPBs by Class I antiarrhythmic drugs (nomenclature by Vaughan Williams), performed worldwide for many years, was very harmful. Today, beta-blockers are generally used, which do not significantly influence the frequency of VPBs, but reduce the risk for sudden death.

Chapter 26
Ventricular Tachycardia

Ventricular tachycardia (VT) is a severe arrhythmia that often impairs heart function considerably and can be a precursor of ventricular fibrillation. Herein, the impact of VT on hemodynamics and prognosis is distinguished. The hemodynamic response to VT depends on the preexisting left ventricular (LV) (or right ventricular) ejection fraction (EF) and the rate and duration of tachycardia. The worse the ventricular function and the faster the rate, the worse the ventricular filling and output are. A long-duration VT (minutes to hours or even days) generally leads to a further hemodynamic deterioration. The prognosis of VT is determined by the kind and severity of the underlying cardiac disease. The pathophysiologic mechanisms are enhanced automaticity, micro-reentry, and triggered activity.

Definition and Characteristics of Ventricular Tachycardia

VT is defined as ≥ 3 consecutive premature ventricular complexes with a QRS duration of >0.12 s (often ≥ 0.14 s) and a rate between 100 to 240 beats/min, exceptionally up to 300 beats/min, but generally 130–220 beats/min. The QRS complexes are not preceded by atrial deflections. The tachycardia may be sustained (duration >30 s, often lasting minutes to hours) or nonsustained (duration <30 s, often shorter) (ECG 26.1). The repolarization is always altered, with ST elevation or depression and T inversion in some leads.

Types of Ventricular Tachycardia

There are three types of VT that generally differ in morphology, clinical significance, and often etiology. These are discussed below.

M. Gertsch, *The ECG Manual: An Evidence-Based Approach*,
© Springer-Verlag London Limited 2009

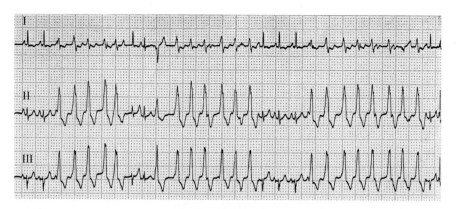

ECG 26.1 Electrocardiogram (ECG) obtained from a 40-year-old woman with palpitations. ECG (leads I, II, III; paper speed 10 mm/s): nonsustained (monomorphic) ventricular tachycardias

Monomorphic Ventricular Tachycardia

Monomorphic VT is the most frequent VT. It may be sustained or nonsustained. Sustained monomorphic VT has a rate of 130–240 beats/min and is initiated by a ventricular premature beat. The tachycardia is regular or minimally irregular. If VT terminates spontaneously, it is followed by a post-tachycardia pause (ECG 26.2a, b), except in atrial fibrillation. Monomorphic VT generally shows a left bundle-branch block (LBBB)-like or right bundle-branch block (RBBB)-like QRS pattern. ECG 26.3a and b show two episodes of VT in a patient with LBBB pattern; ECG 26.3c shows the patient's electrocardiogram (ECG) in sinus rhythm (SR), with an RBBB + LAFB pattern and an extensive anterior myocardial infarction. ECG 26.4a shows an example of VT with an RBBB-like pattern and retrograde atrioventricular (AV) block 2°; ECG 26.4b is the QRS configuration in SR.

A VT with a rate >200 beats/min is called ventricular flutter by some authors. Other authors only use the term ventricular flutter if the morphology of VT is sinusform-like, so that depolarization and repolarization can no longer be distinguished.

AV dissociation, one or more fusion beats, capture beats, or a retrograde AV block 2° (rare) indicate a ventricular origin of the tachycardia in a very high percentage. ECGs 26.4a and 26.5–26.7 demonstrate retrograde AV block 2°.

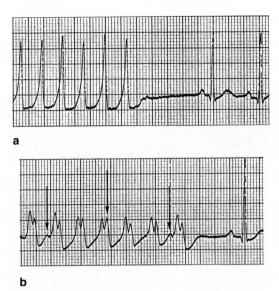

ECG 26.2 Electrocardiogram obtained from a 72-year old man with respiratory insufficiency.
a. Monitor lead (lead II): ventricular tachycardia (VT), rate 220 beats/min. Note the post-tachycardia pause. **b.** Monitor lead: VT, rate 182 beats/min, with different QRS morphology and shorter
post-tachycardia pause. Atrioventricular dissociation: before the second and before the last VT
QRS, a p wave is detectable, and another is hidden within the second (higher) deflection of the
fourth QRS (arrows)

Ventricular capture beats are intermittent supraventricular beats, mostly of sinusal
origin, with a narrow (normal broad) QRS complex. Unfortunately, a retrograde AV
block and fusion beats as well as capture beats are relatively rare phenomena during
VT. Atrial capture means retrograde activation of the atria. It is always present in
supraventricular tachycardia (SVT) and in >60% of VT. However, in VT, the p
waves are mostly not detectable. In nonsustained VT, the QRS complexes may be
monomorphic or more or less polymorphic.

Etiology of Monomorphic Ventricular Tachycardia

The current etiology of monomorphic VT is a coronary heart disease (CHD).
However, all diseases of the LV, and more rarely, diseases of the right ventricle, such
as congenital heart diseases and arrhythmogenic right ventricular dysplasia, can

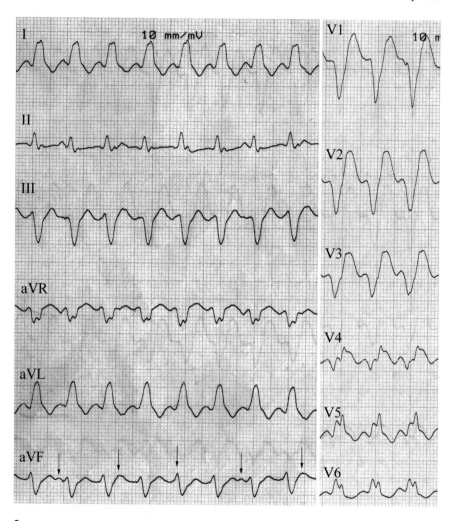

a

ECG 26.3 Electrocardiogram obtained from a 70-year-old man with previous anterior infarction with aneurysm. **a.** Ventricular tachycardia (VT) with a left bundle-branch block (LBBB)-like QRS. QRS duration 160 ms. Ventricular rate 143 beats/min. Atrioventricular dissociation, best recognizable in lead aVF (arrow), atrial rate 85 beats/min. "Nadir" sign in lead V_1 is 90 ms. Note that the transition zone is similar to aberration, with quite abrupt change of negative to positive QRS in V_4/V_5, possibly attributable to previous anterior infarction

provoke this type of VT. It may even be seen in people without an apparent structural heart disease. This special type of tachycardia was formerly called *idiopathic VT*. A substantial number of idiopathic VT invasive electrophysiologic studies have revealed a "focus" in the right ventricular outflow tract, responsible for a typical ECG with LBBB-like pattern and frontal QRS right axis deviation (ECG 26.7). The prognosis of VT depends on the kind and severity of the heart disease.

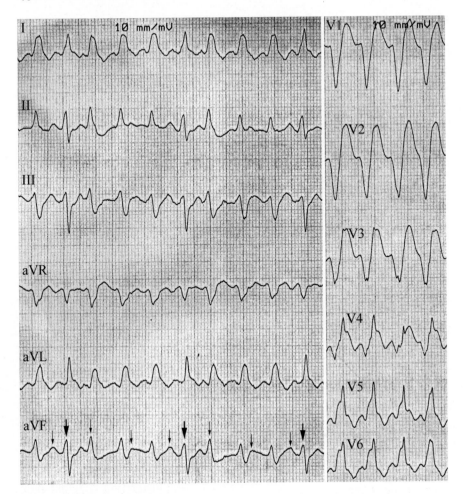

b

ECG 26.3 (continued) **b.** VT with LBBB-like QRS. Ventricular rate 164 beats/min. AV dissociation atrial rate 123 beats/min (small arrows). Fusion beats (big arrows), with shorter duration
and different configuration, preceded by p waves (hidden within the T wave). Another proof for
ventricular origin of the tachycardia is the LBBB-like pattern in this patient with right bundle-
branch block (RBBB) + left anterior fascicular block (LAFB) aberration in sinus rhythm (part c)

ECG 26.3 (continued) **c.** Sinus rhythm (rate 69 beats/min). LAFB + RBBB. Extensive previous anterior infarction, ST elevation (V_2 to V_4) attributable to aneurysm

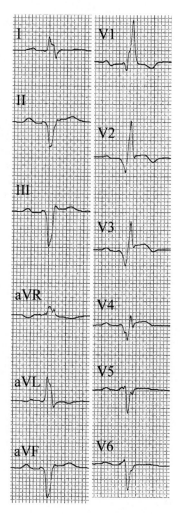

c

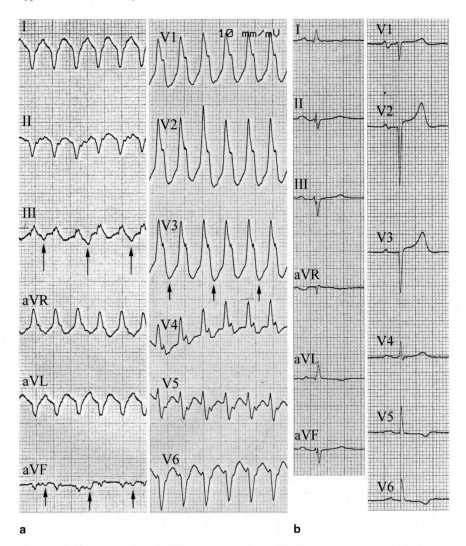

a   b

ECG 26.4 Electrocardiogram obtained from a 76-year-old man with coronary artery disease, history of two unlocalizable infarctions. **a.** Ventricular tachycardia with right bundle-branch block–like QRS. QRS duration 120 ms. Ventricular rate 236 beats/min. Retrograde 2:1 atrioventricular block (2:1 ventriculoatrial block), best detectable in leads III and aVF (arrows), atrial rate 118 beats/min. **b.** Sinus rhythm (rate 65 beats/min). Frontal QRS axis −30°. Peripheral low voltage with slightly notched QRS. Absent R progression in V_1 to V_3. Negative symmetric T waves in V_5/V_6. No distinct infarction pattern

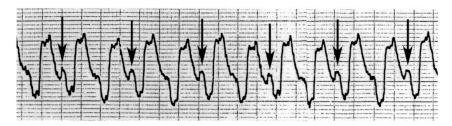

ECG 26.5 Electrocardiogram obtained from an 82-year-old man with coronary heart disease. Monitor lead: ventricular tachycardia, rate 172 beats/min, with retrograde 2:1 atrioventricular block (2:1 ventriculoatrial block) (see arrow)

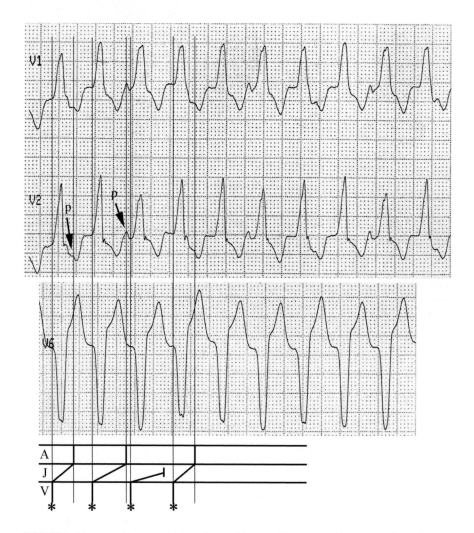

ECG 26.6 Electrocardiogram obtained from a 92-year-old woman with coronary heart disease. Leads V_1/V_2/V_6. Ventricular tachycardia with right bundle-branch–like pattern and QS complex in V_6. Retrograde atrioventricular block 2° type Wenckebach

ECG 26.7 Electrocardiogram (ECG) obtained from a 36-year-old man with presyncope episodes associated with palpitations. ECG: ventricular tachycardia (VT), rate 190 beats/min. Frontal QRS axis +100° and the left bundle-branch–like QRS pattern suggest a VT arising in the right ventricular outflow tract (confirmed by electrophysiologic testing). Note: retrograde atrioventricular block 2:1 (see arrows)

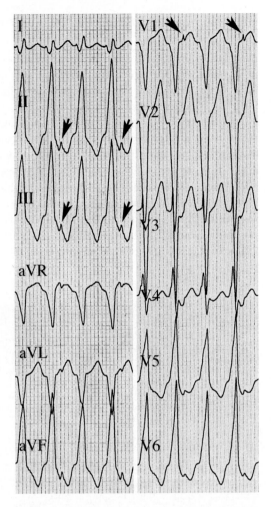

Polymorphic Torsades de Pointes Ventricular Tachycardia

Torsades de pointes VT is characterized by a special ECG morphology. According to the term, the points of the QRS complexes gradually and repetitively change their polarity, "twisting" around the isoelectric line, thus appearing as peaky R and S waves. This peculiarity is often not seen in a single lead. The rate is frequently excessively high—between 200 and 300 beats/min (ECG 26.8), exceptionally up to 400 beats/min (ECG 26.9). A tachycardia of torsades de pointes type in most cases terminates spontaneously after several seconds or even after minutes, despite a high rate. Attacks lasting longer than 5–10 s often lead to loss of consciousness, and a long-lasting tachycardia may provoke organic, especially cerebral damage. However, in relatively rare cases, torsades de pointes tachycardia degenerates into ventricular fibrillation. Because this deleterious complication is not predictable, any patient with this tachycardia should immediately be monitored and treated with magnesium and potassium and/or a pacemaker, with a defibrillator standby.

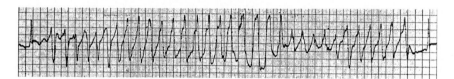

ECG 26.8 Self-limiting polymorphic ventricular tachycardia of the type torsades de pointes, rate approximately 220 beats/min (the first and last beat are normal)

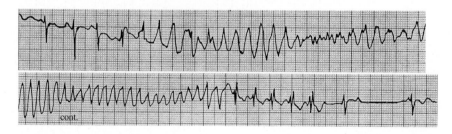

ECG 26.9 Electrocardiogram (ECG) obtained from a 32-year-old woman with anorexia nervosa. Potassium 2.2 mmol/L. ECG (continuous strip): typical ventricular tachycardia (VT) of the type torsades de pointes during 9.5 s, with a maximal rate of 390 beats/min (!), unusually changing into a supraventricular rhythm with right bundle-branch block (or to a regular VT?) at a rate of 176 beats/min, before spontaneous conversion into an atrioventricular (AV) rhythm with AV dissociation, rate approximately 60 beats/min

Etiology of Torsades de Pointes Ventricular Tachycardia

VT of the torsades de pointes type was first associated with the congenital "long QT syndromes," the Romano-Ward syndrome (without deafness), and the Jervell and Lange-Nielson syndrome (with deafness). The acquired long QT is much more frequent and caused by many conditions and agents leading to a prolongation of the QT interval. The most common agents are diuretics (provoking hypokalemia often combined with hypomagnesemia) and antiarrhythmic drugs, especially of Vaughan Williams class Ia. However, torsades de pointes has been observed in many other conditions, such as CHD with and without bradycardia, and by many other drugs.

Polymorphic Ventricular Tachycardia

In many publications, the term "polymorphic" refers only to polymorphic VT of the torsade de pointes type. However, there are polymorphic VTs without torsades de pointes:

1. Polymorphous QRS complexes are not uncommon in nonsustained VT, especially if the tachycardia only lasts for several beats.
2. Polymorphy of the QRS complexes without torsades de pointes is occasionally seen in patients with severe myocardial damage and is associated with a poor prognosis. The rate is often not excessive (ECG 26.10), but degeneration into ventricular fibrillation is common. This VT type can also be observed in patients with cardiogenic shock shortly before death.

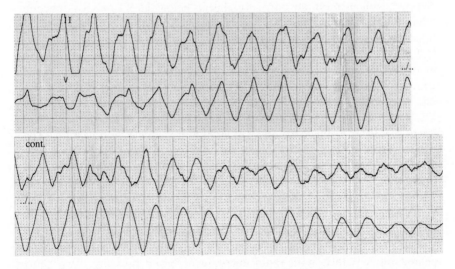

ECG 26.10 Electrocardiogram (ECG) obtained from a 97-year-old man with terminal heart failure. ECG (continuous monitor strip): after two slow beats, polymorphic ventricular tachycardia without torsades de pointes. Rate approximately 130 beats/min

A Special Condition: Accelerated Idioventricular Rhythm

Accelerated idioventricular rhythm is not a VT, by definition, because its rate rarely exceeds 100 beats/min. However, it does not represent an escape rhythm (as in the case of a low-rate ventricular rhythm in complete AV block) and therefore is often not clearly identified. In most cases, a ventricular rhythm (with broad QRS) arises during several beats, generally 2–10, suppressing the SR by a slightly higher rate. At the beginning and end of the ventricular rhythm, fusion beats might be observed.

Accelerated idioventricular rhythm is seen especially in acute myocardial infarction in a high percentage during the first hours after successful thrombolysis, and shortly after coronary bypass operations and is therefore accepted as a reliable marker of myocardial ischemia. As the following case report demonstrates, it can be difficult to classify a VT, and a VT might require an unconventional therapy.

Short Story/Case Report

In 1989, on a Saturday morning, a 54-year-old male patient with a history of two myocardial infarctions was hospitalized because of left heart failure that was confirmed by clinical findings and x-rays. Blood pressure was 90/70 mmHg. The ECG showed a monomorphic VT with a relatively slow rate of 120 beats/min (ECG 26.11a). In a retrospective analysis, AV dissociation could be detected, with an atrial rate only several beats below the VT rate. LV function seemed to be severely impaired (M-mode echo). The VT responded neither to lidocaine nor to amiodarone, intravenously. In another attempt to restore SR, five direct current (DC) shocks were applied, without success. On Monday morning, the general state had dramatically impaired, the patient was in shock with anuria, blood pressure was 70/50 mmHg, the arrhythmia persisted at a rate of about 120 beats/min, now for 48 hours. The story of this relatively slow VT, unresponsive to antiarrhythmic drugs and DC shock, was rediscussed and it was decided to evaluate the effect of atrial overpacing as "ultima ratio." The cardiac index (determined by thermodilution) was 3.1L/m^2. Right atrial pacing was successful at a rate several beats above the VT rate, with a PQ interval of 0.2 s and a bundle-branch block pattern (ECG 26.11b). In the following 20 min, blood pressure slowly increased to 100/70 mmHg, the cardiac index increased to 4.2L/m^2, and the patient was more alert. The cardiac state stabilized under constant atrial pacing, and 4 hours later diuresis recovered. During repetitive short interruption of pacing, VT at a rate of 120 beats/min reappeared immediately, with rapid decrease of blood pressure. Two short episodes of sinus tachycardia at a rate of 120–122 beats/min were also observed. Sixteen hours later, the arrhythmia stopped, without antiarrhythmic drug. Coronary angiography revealed severe three-vessel disease and an LV EF of 30%. The patient was operated on the next day (four bypasses), recovered definitively, and was still alive 9 years later.

In conclusion, in this patient with severe CHD, cardiogenic (arrhythmogenic) shock was reversible by atrial overpacing of a low-rate VT, an apparently life-saving procedure. The VT could be classified as a relatively slow "common" monomorphic VT or as accelerated idioventricular rhythm, extremely atypical in duration and high rate. The VT, unresponsive to drugs and electroconversion, supports the latter diagnosis.

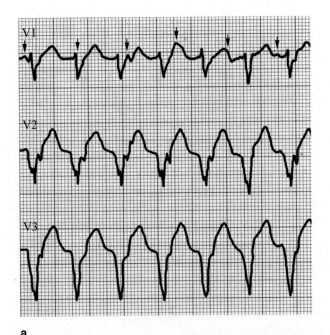

a

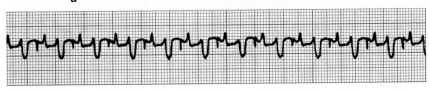

b

ECG 26.11 Electrocardiogram obtained from a 53-year-old man, described in the Short Story. **a.** Accelerated idioventricular rhythm, rate 120 beats/min. Atrioventricular dissociation detectable in lead V_1 (arrow) **b.** Atrial overpacing at a rate of 122 beats/min (monitor lead)

Other Rare Types of Ventricular Tachycardia

VT types such as fascicular tachycardias and bidirectional tachycardias are extremely rare.

Differential Diagnosis of Wide-QRS Tachycardias: Ventricular Tachycardia Versus Supraventricular Tachycardia with Aberration

Not only VTs, but also SVTs with aberration (SVTab), lead to broad QRS complexes ($\geq 0.12\,s$).

Types of Supraventricular Tachycardia with Aberration (Wide QRS)

Three types of SVTab are distinguished.

Supraventricular Tachycardia with Aberration with Bundle-Branch Block

SVTs such as atrial flutter, atrial fibrillation, AV tachycardia, and sinus tachycardia with or without detectable p waves with bundle-branch block (rarely bilateral bundle-branch block) represent the most common forms of SVTab with wide QRS. In all cases of wide QRS tachycardias at a moderate rate (110–150 beats/min), a sinus tachycardia with bundle-branch block aberration should be excluded. The p wave may be hidden within the T wave of the preceding beat, especially in the presence of a long PQ interval.

Supraventricular Tachycardia with Aberration in Wolff-Parkinson-White Syndrome

This rare condition only occurs by conduction antegradely through the accessory pathway, or in cases of additional bundle-branch block. More than 90% of the "Wolff-Parkinson-White tachycardia" show a narrow, normal QRS.

Supraventricular Tachycardia with Other Aberration

In some textbooks, a third type of SVTab is mentioned, to provide a category for an unidentifiable aberration that is neither connected with bundle-branch block (bilateral block included) nor with the Wolff-Parkinson-White syndrome. It has to be mentioned that, in rare cases, a wide QRS can be present without aberration, for instance in severe ventricular hypertrophy and in myocardial infarction.

Differentiating Between Ventricular Tachycardia and Supraventricular Tachycardia with Aberration

Many morphologic ECG criteria have been published concerning alterations of the QRS complex that should allow the differentiation between VT and SVTab. The common characteristics are summarized in Table 26.1. However, even experienced

Table 26.1 ECG differentiation between VT and SVTab

VT	SVTab
• AV dissociation	• No AV dissociation
• Fusion beats	• Rarely fusion beats in WPW tachycardia
• Retrograde AV block (VA block) 2° (2:1 block or Wenckebach)	• No VA block 2°
QRS:	
• Purely negative QRS in V_1 to V_6	• Never seen in SVTab
• Purely positive QRS in V_1 to V_6	• Only in antidromic WPW tachycardia
• QRS amplitude strikingly high	• Very high QRS amplitude only in rare cases of WPW tachycardia
• QRS duration ≥160 ms	• QRS ≥160 ms only in severe LVH, RVH, or hyperkalemia
• Superior QRS axis	• Other than superior QRS axis (exception: LAFB)
• In presence of BBB pattern in SR: different BBB pattern during tachycardia	• In presence of BBB pattern in SR: identical BBB pattern in tachycardia
• QRS in VT similar to VPB in SR—unreliable	
LBBB-like morphology	
• "NADIR sign" ≥70 ms (lead V_1/V_2)	• "NADIR sign" ≤60 ms
• Q wave in lead V_6	• No Q wave in lead V_6
RBBB-like morphology	
• QS configuration in leads V_6 and aVF	• No QS in V_6 and aVF
• Mono- or biphasic QRS in lead V_1(R, QR, RS)—unreliable	• Any QRS configuration in V_1. *Note*: A rsR′ type strongly favors SVT!
Note: The signs for VT are highly specific but show low sensitivity!	*Note*: Several signs for SVTab do not exclude VT!

ECG, electrocardiogram; VT, ventricular tachycardia; SVTab, supraventricular tachycardia with aberration; AV, atrioventricular; WPW, Wolff-Parkinson-White; VA, ventriculoatrial; LVH, left ventricular hypertrophy; RVH, right ventricular hypertrophy; BBB, bundle-branch block; VPB, ventricular premature beat; SR, sinus rhythm; LAFB, left anterior fascicular block; LBBB, left bundle-branch block; RBBB, right bundle-branch block.

rhythmologists only reach a 85% accuracy, even if all 12 standard leads are available. Those readers who have neither the time nor would enjoy learning all these rather complicated morphologic ECG signs may resort to a more simple approach.

Tchou et al. [Tchou P, Young P, Mahmud R, et al. Useful clinical criteria for the diagnosis of ventricular tachycardia. Am J Med 1988;84:53–56] found that 29 of the 31 patients they studied (aged 27–79 years, 10 women), almost all with myocardial infarction, with broad QRS tachycardias proven with electrophysiologic studies, had VT, whereas the clinical (visual) diagnosis before was VT in 17 and SVTab in 14 patients. All patients with proven VT had experienced symptoms related to tachycardia after a recent myocardial infarction. However, it is obvious that this "rule" is valid only in this condition.

Differentiating Between Ventricular Tachycardia and Artifacts

Artifacts can be misdiagnosed as wide complex tachycardias, especially in rhythm strips. Generally, these artifacts are attributable to mechanical maneuvers such as teeth-brushing, knocking on the back during physiotherapy, or, rarely, insufficient skin/electrode contact. A careful analysis of the ECG allows the identification of remnant QRS complexes (so-called "notches") within the artifacts (ECG 26.12) and also an atypical beginning and end of the "artifact VT."

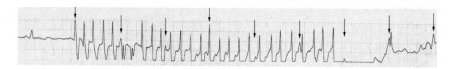

ECG 26.12 Continuous strip. Pseudo–ventricular tachycardia. Artifacts during teeth-brushing. Rate up to >300 beats/min. The basic rhythm (sinus rhythm) is slightly irregular (arrow, indicating "notches" that are scarcely visible). However, the too-narrow "R waves," the excessive rate, and additional artifacts, for instance the shift of the curve off the paper, clearly indicate artifacts

Therapy for Ventricular Tachycardia

As mentioned above, differentiation between VT and SVTab can be difficult or even impossible on the basis of the ECG. However, it is extremely important to make the true diagnosis *before* drug treatment. Misdiagnosis of a wide QRS tachycardia as SVTab, in the presence of VT, could result in life-threatening complications. For example: A VT is misdiagnosed as SVT with bundle-branch block aberration and treated with verapamil or another cardiodepressive drug, intravenously. The tachycardia does not respond, but blood pressure decreases dramatically and leads to death.

Moreover, some antiarrhythmic drugs impair the effect of external DC conversion. In all unclear cases, DC conversion is the only correct therapy! Of course, oxygen should be applied and cardiodepressive narcotics must be avoided. In the presence of VT, lidocaine is only successful in 20%–30% of cases, and procainamide, which produces a decrease in systolic blood pressure of 10–20 mmHg or more, is only successful in approximately 80% of cases.

In summary, a wide QRS complex tachycardia at a high rate often needs immediate DC conversion. Unprofessional "pre-treating" with antiarrhythmic drugs may not only be deleterious in itself, but could impair or inhibit the success of DC conversion.

Chapter 27
Pacemaker Electrocardiogram

The first implantable cardiac stimulator device was applied in humans in 1958. Since its introduction, this ingenious method for treating bradycardiac arrhythmias has spread worldwide. In 1998 alone, 601,000 new pacemakers were implanted. The total number of patients with a pacemaker is estimated to be more than 8 million. In a world population of more than 8 billion, that is approximately 1 in 1000 people.

The first pacemaker, implanted by Senning in 1958, was fixed rate, without sensing of spontaneous heart beats. The next steps in pacemaker evolution were the "on-demand device" (with sensing of spontaneous rhythm), the double-chamber pacemaker [allowing an atrioventricular (AV) sequential pacing], and the rate-responsive device that accelerates the pacing rate by analyzing body movement, respiration rate, and other parameters. In recent years, additional sophisticated functions have been integrated, such as mode switch (automatic change from two-chamber pacing to ventricular pacing after the onset of atrial fibrillation), sleep function, telemetry including memory properties for counts of spontaneous and paced beats in detail, and programmed rapid atrial stimulation.

Morphologic Features of the Pacemaker Electrocardiogram

More than 98% of the pacemakers are implanted transvenously through the subclavian vein, with the electrode in the right ventricle (RV). In approximately 30% of patients with a pacemaker, an atrial electrode in the right atrium is implanted additionally. In common ventricular pacing, the RV is activated first and the left ventricle (LV) with latency over the septum, leading to a left bundle-branch block (LBBB) pattern. De- and repolarization are uniform in the limb leads, with broad R waves in leads I and aVL and wide QS complexes in leads II, aVF, and III. In the precordial leads, we mainly miss a positive QRS deflection in leads V_5/V_6 as frequently seen in LBBB aberration in a supraventricular rhythm. In most cases, after the stimulation spike, we observe a QS complex in V_1 to V_5 and an rS complex in V_6. Because of a special position of the ventricular lead within the RV, the rare pattern of Rs in lead V_1 may be detectable, a pattern never seen in LBBB aberration.

M. Gertsch, *The ECG Manual: An Evidence-Based Approach,*
© Springer-Verlag London Limited 2009

In the remaining 2% of patients, with, for example, a single-ventricle, severe tri-cuspid incompetence (if a screw-in electrode was not considered), the electrode is attached at the epicardium of the LV by the surgeon. In this case, the LV is activated before the RV, resulting in a more or less typical right bundle-branch block (RBBB) pattern. Patterns of previous myocardial infarction are easily detectable in the rare conditions of epicardial LV pacing with RBBB pattern, but not in the majority of patients with endocardial RV pacing and with an LBBB pattern. A broad Q or QS wave in the inferior and anteroseptal leads, not uncommon in RV pacing with an LBBB pattern, may also imitate an infarction pattern. The QRS complex is wide, however. Pacemaker spikes are of greater amplitude in unipolar pacing compared with bipolar pacing. The spike can be so small that it is overlooked, especially in a generator output of 2.0–2.50 V.

One-Chamber Pacemaker

The electrocardiogram (ECG) pattern depends on the rate of the pacemaker on one hand, and on the spontaneous heart rate on the other hand. If the artificial pacing rate is higher than the spontaneous rate, every heart beat is paced.

The electric stimulus is mediated by the electrode that is localized in the RV. The RV is activated first and the LV over the septum, with latency. Consequently, an LBBB pattern is seen in the ECG (ECG 27.1). In the rare cases of left ventricular pacing (through an electrode attached on the surface of the LV), an RBBB pattern results. The electric stimulus itself manifests as small and short spikes immediately before the QRS complex. The stimulus is positive, negative, biphasic, or not visible, depending on its projection to the lead (ECG 27.1). Unipolar pacing results in markedly higher spikes than bipolar pacing.

The sensing mechanism of a pacemaker ("on-demand function") inhibits pacing during and shortly after one or several premature beats (ECG 27.2). Equally, the pacer function is inhibited if the pacing rate is lower than the spontaneous rhythm over a longer period. Thus, there is no sign in the ECG that would identify the patient as having a pacemaker. It is possible in these cases to switch the on-demand mode to a fixed-rate mode with a magnet placed on the skin above the generator (ECG 27.3).

In cases with nearly the same rate of the pacemaker and the spontaneous rhythm, fusion beats or pseudo-fusion beats are detectable. In a fusion beat, the ventricles are partially activated by the pacer and partially activated spontaneously (ECGs 27.4 and 27.5). In a pseudo-fusion beat, the stimulus occurs too late during the absolute refractory ventricular period and remains ineffective—the heart is exclu-sively activated spontaneously (ECGs 27.4 and 27.5). Fusion beats and pseudo-fusion beats are normal features in a pacemaker ECG.

ECG 27.1 Electrocardiogram (ECG) obtained from an
82-year-old woman with bradycardic atrial fibrillation
(mean rate 30 beats/min), presyncope. ECG: VVI(R)
pacemaker, rate 70 beats/min (at rest). Every spike is followed
by a wide QRS complex with left bundle-branch block
pattern (endocardial right ventricular pacing). Atrial fibrillation. Note the different polarity of the pacemaker spikes
(positive, negative, biphasic) in different leads

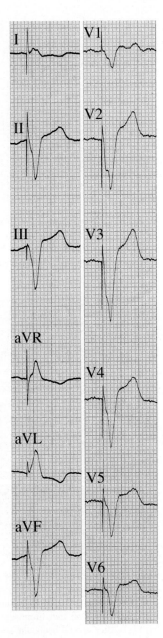

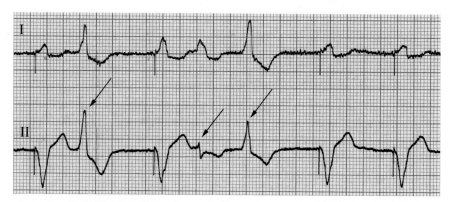

ECG 27.2 Electrocardiogram (ECG) obtained from a 74-year-old woman with complete atrioventricular block, atrial fibrillation. ECG: VVI pacemaker, rate 70 beats/min. The pacemaker senses the (ventricular) premature beats (arrows) and pacing only occurs after an escape interval that nearly corresponds to the pacing rate

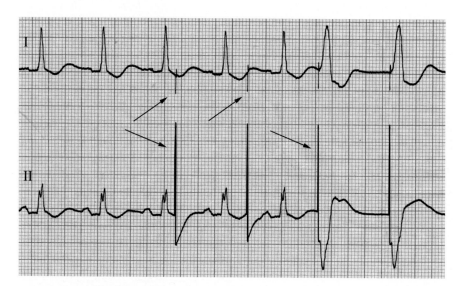

ECG 27.3 Electrocardiogram (ECG) obtained from an 80-year-old man with sick sinus syndrome (with intermittent sinus arrest, not shown). VVI pacemaker (1974). ECG: sinus rhythm, rate 82 beats/min. After positioning a magnet, the pacemaker delivers impulses at a rate of 71 beats/min. The first two impulses are ineffective because they fall into the refractory period (arrows). After several beats, the sinus node takes over the heart action again (not shown)

The pacing rate varies in all patients with a rate responsive device, depending on the current activity. In general, the pacemaker rate is programmed to a maximal rate of 150 beats/min and a minimal rate of 60 beats/min. These pacing devices are called VVI(R) (rate responsiveness in ventricular pacing).

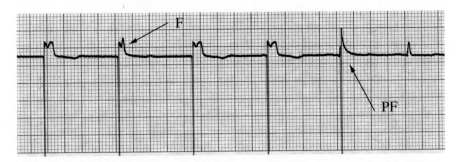

ECG 27.4 Electrocardiogram (ECG) obtained from a 77-year-old man with sick sinus syndrome. VVI pacemaker (implanted in 1972). ECG: Because of nearly the same rate of the pacemaker and the sinus node, the rhythms often change. The second beat is a fusion beat ($\downarrow$F), the fifth beat is a pseudo-fusion beat ($\uparrow$PF)

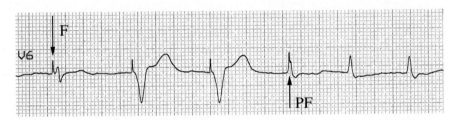

ECG 27.5 Electrocardiogram (ECG) obtained from an 86-year-old man with bradycardic atrial fibrillation, presyncope. VVI(R) pacemaker. ECG: Change between conducted and paced beats. One fusion beat ($\downarrow$F), one pseudo-fusion beat ($\downarrow$PF)

Double-Chamber Pacemaker

This device consists of a ventricular electrode in the RV and an additional electrode in the right atrium, allowing sequential AV pacing. The right atrium (and the left atrium shortly after) is only paced if the spontaneous atrial rate is lower than the pacing rate. As in ventricular pacing, in atrial pacing a pacemaker spike is visible, in this case at the beginning of the p wave. ECG 27.6 shows AV sequential double-chamber pacing. In ECG 27.7, there is spontaneous activation of the atria by the sinus stimulus because the sinus rate is higher than the atrial rate of the pacemaker. Therefore, the atrial spike is lacking. In both conditions (ECGs 27.6 and 27.7), the ventricles are activated by the pacemaker.

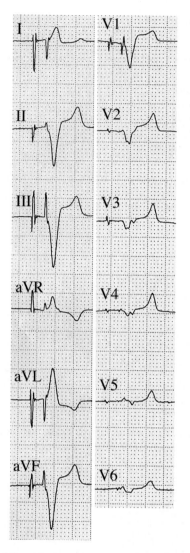

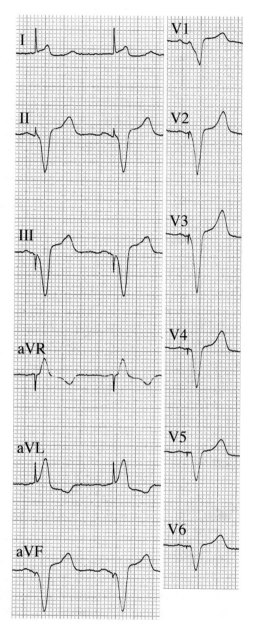

ECG 27.6 Electrocardiogram (ECG) obtained from a 55-year-old woman with complete atrioventricular (AV) block and sinus node dysfunction. DDD(R) pacemaker. ECG: AV sequential pacing of the atrium and the ventricle, at a rate of 70 beats/min. Note the pacemaker spikes before the (flat) p waves and QRS complexes

ECG 27.7 Electrocardiogram (ECG) obtained from a 62-year-old man with sick sinus syndrome. DDD(R) pacemaker. ECG: The p waves are sensed and the ventricles stimulated atrioventricularly sequentially, at the sinusal rate of 67 beats/min in limb leads and 72 beats/min in precordial leads

Electric Complications and Failures

There are manifold generator and electrode complications with pacemakers. There are early complications that occur immediately after implantation, and later complications that occur 5–8 years after implantation.

The early complications mainly result from electrode displacement or incorrect connection of the electrode to the generator (not as rare as one would expect). These complications, leading to loss of capture, are generally recognized during the postoperative period in the hospital and need immediate revision.

The late complications that occur after several years are provoked either by depletion of the battery or critical increase of the stimulation threshold, or both. Both conditions lead to loss of capture. Beginning battery depletion is announced by decrease of the stimulation rate and/or change to the fixed-rate mode. In many cases of advanced depletion, the pacemaker spike is still visible in the ECG, but without consecutive QRS complex (ECG 27.8). In dual-chamber dual-inhibited (DDD) pacemaker ECGs, beginning battery depletion is characterized by a change of DDD function to VVO function, at a decreased pacing rate. ECG 27.9 shows intermittent pacemaker failure during pacemaker implantation, and ECG 27.10 shows intermittent nonfunction caused by a manipulation during pacemaker control. In cases of battery depletion, the generator must be replaced immediately. Fortunately, the favorable time for replacement of the generator can be estimated in advance with an accuracy of about 1 month. Most pacemaker control devices automatically indicate the lifetime of a generator battery. At the same time, the current pacing threshold is measured. A loss of capture can also occur during threshold measurement if the output of the pacemaker is decreased below the current threshold. However, in pacemaker-dependent patients, a long ventricular pause (ECG 27.10) should be avoided.

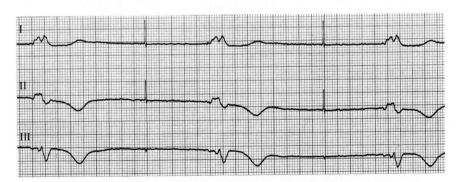

ECG 27.8 Electrocardiogram (ECG) obtained from a 75-year-old man with complete atrioventricular block, atrial fibrillation. Generator depletion of a VVI pacemaker. ECG (50 mm/s): ineffective pacemaker spikes (decreased rate of 44 beats/min). Ventricular escape rhythm. Rate 44 beats/min. The sensing function is still in action. The f waves are not visible in these leads

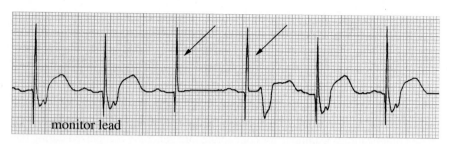

ECG 27.9 Electrocardiogram (ECG) obtained from a 60-year-old woman with sick sinus syndrome, atrioventricular block 1°. The ECG (monitor lead) during implantation of a DDD pacemaker shows intermittent pacemaker dysfunction, caused by unstable position of the electrode tip. Two ventricular spikes are ineffective; the spontaneous sinus beats with pseudo-fusion (↓) are not sensed

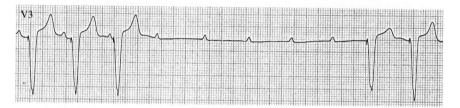

ECG 27.10 Electrocardiogram (ECG) obtained from a 64-year-old woman with complete atrioventricular block, Morgagni-Adams-Stokes attacks. VVI pacemaker. ECG: During pacemaker control, the pacemaker was inadvertently inhibited for several seconds. A ventricular asystole of 4.2 s occurred, without symptoms

Complications between the early and the late stages are relatively rare and generally include other situations. Unexpected premature battery depletion or a critical increase of the threshold have become rare complications at this stage. The main intermediate complications are discussed in the following two paragraphs.

Undersensing and Oversensing

In undersensing, the programmed sensing level (in mV) of the generator is too high (too insensitive) for the normal sensing of the spontaneous QRS complex. Therefore, the pacer runs in a "fixed-rate mode." This can occur constantly or in isolated beats only. The ECG is characterized by spikes falling into the spontaneous cardiac cycle at random (ECG 27.11). Ventricular spikes falling into the refractory ventricular period of the spontaneous ventricular cycle do not, of course, result in stimulated beats and can visually simulate a loss of capture. The same could occur with atrial spikes in respect to atrial cycles. Undersensing could theoretically be a dangerous situation. A spike falling into the potential vulnerable period of the ventricle (spike on T phenomenon) might induce ventricular fibrillation. However,

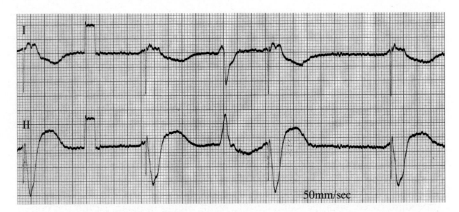

ECG 27.11 Electrocardiogram (ECG) obtained from an 82-year-old man with complete atrioventricular block. VVI pacemaker. ECG (50 mm/s): ventricular pacing, rate 69 beats/min. The ventricular premature beat is not sensed (undersensing)

this extremely rare complication probably occurs only in patients with severe ischemia. In practice, undersensing is harmless and does not induce symptoms.

Undersensing is eliminated by lowering the sensing threshold, e.g., from 2.5 to 1.5 mV. This represents a more or less cosmetic procedure, because complications (e.g., ventricular fibrillation because of the pacemaker spike falling into the vulnerable period of the ventricular premature beat) are extremely rare. Moreover, sensing-threshold lowering may induce oversensing, which leads more often to dangerous situations.

In oversensing, the programmed sensing level is too low (too sensitive). Thus, small electric forces, mainly arising in the upper thoracic skeleton muscles (pectoralis major, sternocleidomastoideus) are sensed, leading to inhibition of the pacemaker. In some cases, inhibition lasts several heart cycles and can lead to syncope in a currently pacemaker-dependent patient. The corresponding ECG might be detected in an ambulatory ECG and is characterized by multiple small spikes produced by skeletal muscles, absent pacemaker spikes, and ventricular asystole (ECG 27.12). Because oversensing preferentially occurs during extreme

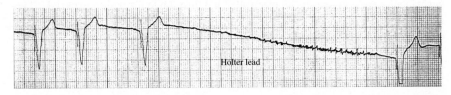

ECG 27.12 Electrocardiogram (ECG) obtained from a 65-year-old man with complete atrioventricular block, syncope. Presyncope after VVI pacemaker implantation (1976), while chopping wood. ECG (Holter lead): The great pacemaker spikes suggest unipolar pacing. The third paced beat arises with small latency (inhibited for a very short period), then ventricular asystole occurs during 5 s. The inhibiting muscle potentials are scarcely visible. Oversensing and the symptoms disappeared after programming the sensitivity from 2.5 to 5.0 mV

stress of these muscles, correlated activities, such as chopping wood in younger patients or leaving the bathtub in older patients, a dangerous situation could arise, including the loss of consciousness (see Short Story).

Short Story/Case Report

In 1978, a 79-year-old patient with a VVI pacemaker, implanted for complete AV block with syncopal attacks, wanted to leave the bathtub, still full of water. He heaved himself up with his arms and lost consciousness. When he awoke, he lay again in the bathtub, with his head partially under water. He repeated the procedure twice, with the same terrible result. Being in panic, he did not consider draining off the water. With an extreme effort, he catapulted himself out of the bathtub. Again he lost consciousness. But then he realized with great satisfaction that he was lying on the floor, outside of the bathtub.

The control of the pacemaker revealed oversensing, reproducible by strong strain of the arm and thoracic muscles, with consecutive cardiac arrest during several seconds. The patient was enthusiastic about this test and asked for repetitions, up to short loss of consciousness. After changing the sensitivity of the pacemaker from 2.5 to 4 mV (the R wave reading was 7.4 mV), the patient remained free of symptoms.

Oversensing mainly occurs in patients with unipolar electrodes, where the sensed area is considerably greater than in bipolar electrodes. Oversensing has become rare because of the better sensing properties of the pacemakers, distinguishing more precisely between heart potentials and skeletal muscle potentials. Oversensing is eliminated by increasing the sensing threshold, e.g., from 2 to 4 mV.

Lead Fracture, Lead Insulation Damage

Lead fracture and lead insulation damages can occur as a result of accidents, permanent wear and tear of the electrode, and unsuitable insulation materials. The most current and dangerous result is a loss of capture. Electrode damages are often detectable in changes of lead parameters before a loss of capture arises.

Control of Pacemaker Patients

Out-hospital general practitioners and specialists in internal medicine and even cardiology generally control only a few pacemaker patients. Pacemaker patients are regularly followed up in the hospital by a specialized team. Because of the vast variability of pacemaker generators, the complexity of control devices of different manufacturers, and the complexity of pacemaker arrhythmias, the members of this team are obliged to undergo continuous education, regularly taking special courses organized by the National Associations of Cardiology and by the manufacturers. Moreover, it is imperative to regularly consult the leading journals in this field, such as *PACE* (edited since 1978) and the *Journal of Cardiovascular Electrophysiology* (since 1989), which reflect the constantly evolving progress in this field. A detailed presentation and discussion of the problems concerning pacemakers, all complex pacemaker arrhythmias included, would go beyond the scope of this book.

Pacemaker Codes

Because of the development of simple one-chamber pacemakers to the current complex devices, a pacemaker code was required for quick identification of the different functions. This code underwent several modifications during the last decades, which reflect the progress. Every cardiologist implanting and controlling pacemakers is familiar with the current code shown in Table 27.1.

Today DDD, DDD(R), VVI, and VVI(R) are the frequently implanted pacing devices. Only dual-chamber pacemakers guarantee AV sequential pacing, with one exception. In atrial-inhibited atrial (AAI) pacing, the atrium is sensed and the ventricle is paced, also resulting in so-called physiologic pacing. Theoretically, VVI or VVI(R) devices should only be implanted in patients with atrial fibrillation, where atrial sensing or pacing is not possible. However, one-chamber ventricular pacing has not yet been abandoned worldwide, on one hand for economic reasons, on the

Table 27.1 The revised NASPE/BPEG generic code for antibradycardia pacing

	Position				
	I	II	III	IV	V
Category	Chamber(s) paced	Chamber(s) sensed	Response to sensing	Rate modulation	Multisite pacing
	O = none	O = none	O = none	O = none	O = none
	A = atrium	A = atrium	T = triggered	R = rate modulation	A = atrium
	V = ventricle	V = ventricle	I = inhibited		V = ventricle
	D = dual	D = dual	D = dual		D = dual
	(A + V)	(A + V)	(T + I)		(A + V)
Manufacturers' designation only	S = single (A or V)	S = single (A or V)			

NASPE, North American Society of Pacing and Electrophysiology; BPEG, British Pacing and Electrophysiology Group.

other because the enthusiasm about the advantages of two-chamber pacing over one-chamber pacing has considerably decreased during the last years. Several important prospective randomized studies have definitively shown that long-term survival and the incidence of cerebral stroke and atrial fibrillation are equal in patients with one-chamber pacemakers compared with those with dual-chamber pacemakers. A significant difference in favor of double-chamber pacing could only be found in patients with sick sinus syndrome in reference to life quality, partly because of the absence of symptoms caused by the pacemaker syndrome.

Pacemaker Syndrome

Prevalence

The prevalence of the syndrome depends on its definition. The prevalence in patients with isolated ventricular pacing is approximately 2% if only serious symptoms are considered, and approximately 22% if all symptoms possibly related to the pacemaker syndrome are considered.

Condition

The pacemaker syndrome is not necessarily linked to VVI(R) pacing. It can also arise in patients with inappropriately programmed AAI(R) or double-chamber pacing. In AAI(R) pacing, AV dyssynchrony can result from a disproportionate increase of the atrial rate during exercise. VDD(R) pacing can lead to the syndrome if the atrial rate decreases below the lower programmed rate resulting in VVI(R) pacing. In DDI(R) pacing, the pacemaker syndrome arises if the spontaneous sinus rate exceeds the lower rate or sensor-indicated rate in patients with AV block because of continual AV dissociation. Even in DDD pacing, prolonged intraatrial and/or interatrial conduction times as well as pacemaker-mediated or endless loop tachycardia can induce AV dyssynchrony or ventriculoatrial synchrony, respectively. A pacemaker syndrome is easily overlooked in these conditions.

Pathophysiologic Mechanisms

The basis of the pacemaker syndrome is the abnormal timing of the atrial and ventricular contraction. The pathophysiologic mechanisms are more complex than formerly assumed. The absence of the atrial kick generally reduces arterial pressure at a modest degree. The atrial contraction against the closed AV valves could result in very high venous a (atrial) waves, up to 50 mmHg. These a waves can provoke an abnormal and exaggerated answer of baroreceptors in the lung veins resulting in a drastic decrease of blood pressure, with a syncope as possible consequence. In recent times, multiple reflex pathways have been postulated to be involved, including carotid and aortic baroreceptors, cardiopulmonary baroreflexes, and others.

Indications for Pacing

The indications for implantation of cardiac pacemakers (and other antiarrhythmic devices) are presented in the 1998 American College of Cardiology/American Heart Association Guidelines with a differentiation into three classes. Class I indication includes conditions for which there is evidence and/or general agreement that a given procedure or treatment is beneficial, useful, and effective. Class II includes conditions with conflicting evidence and/or divergence of opinion about the usefulness/efficacy of treatment. Class III describes conditions with evidence/general opinion that a procedure/treatment is not useful/effective and in some cases could be harmful. The review provides an extensive and detailed allocation of nearly all conditions to the three classes, 333 references included. Thus, only a short overview is presented and two relatively new and interesting indications are discussed.

Complete AV block and sinus node dysfunction (sick sinus syndrome) represent the most frequent reasons for chronic pacing, each of which is responsible for approximately 40% of all pacemaker implantations. The remaining 20% are covered by bradycardiac atrial fibrillation, so-called "prophylactic" implantations in some forms of bifascicular and incomplete trifascicular block (Chapter 11), AV block 2° of Mobitz type or high degree, and by rare conditions such as carotis sinus syndrome, long QT syndrome, sleep apnea, some cases of hypertrophic obstructive cardiomyopathy, and heart failure in patients with wide QRS complexes.

Pacing in Hypertrophic Obstructive Cardiomyopathy

Double-chamber pacing was applied in an attempt to avoid myectomy by open heart surgery. Shortening of the AV interval leads to better LV filling and consecutively to a significant reduction (up to 50%) of the intraventricular systolic gradient and significant improvement of symptoms. During recent years, the so-called transcoronary alcohol septal ablation has proven to be almost as effective as a surgical septal resection. Ethyl ablation provokes necrosis of a portion of the hypertrophic interventricular septum with a dramatic reduction of the gradient, with a latency of several weeks. Surgical resection results in an LBBB, whereas alcohol ablation provokes an RBBB in all cases and complete AV block in >40%. Approximately 20% of the patients need a dual-chamber pacemaker.

Pacing in Heart Failure

A prolonged QRS duration (>0.12 s) contributes to an additional impairment of ventricular function in patients with heart failure, by dyssynchronous ventricular contraction. It has been shown that synchronous pacing of the RV (through a conventionally positioned electrode) and the LV (through an electrode in the coronary sinus and in a coronary vein, thus stimulating the LV from the epicardium) not only shortens the QRS duration but also improves ventricular function. The method is effectual in patients with LBBB and astonishingly also in patients with RBBB. Recent studies diminish exaggerated hope on this method.

Pacemaker-Mediated Arrhythmias

Pacemaker-related arrhythmias include a vast number of arrhythmias, which may be complex, especially in dual-chamber pacemakers. Analyzing those arrhythmias requires the knowledge of the technical properties of a generator and its present programming.

Chapter 28
Congenital and Acquired-Valvular Heart Diseases

Up to the introduction of heart catheterization in the late 1950s, congenital heart disease was diagnosed by the interpretation of symptoms, heart auscultation, thoracic x-rays, and the electrocardiogram (ECG). In 1967, Burch and DePasquale published a 773-page book, *Electrocardiography in the Diagnosis of Congenital Heart Diseases*, in which four forms of single ventricle were diagnosed (or supposed) on the basis of ECG features. However, today, the diagnosis of congenital and acquired heart anomalies is made or proven by heart catheterization and angiography, and even more often, by echocardiogram and color Doppler.

Congenital Heart Diseases

Today, we rarely meet adult patients who have not had surgical correction of their disease. The majority of operated patients reveal the pattern of complete right bundle-branch block (RBBB), as a result of incision of the right ventricle (which produces an equal pattern of RBBB to that caused by proximal block of the right bundle branch).

Atrial Septal Defect of the Ostium Secundum Type

Atrial septal defect of the ostium secundum type (ASD II) is the most frequent congenital heart disease (14%–21%) of all significant congenital heart diseases. In patients with significant left to right shunt (>50%), the ECG is quite uniform, in approximately 90% of the cases (ECG 28.1):

1. Frontal QRS axis ($\mathring{A}QRS_F$) approximately +60°
2. Incomplete RBBB (iRBBB), generally with an r' > r
3. Slight clockwise rotation, especially in patients with markedly dilated right ventricle (RV)
4. T wave negativity in V_2 (eventually up to V_4/V_5)

M. Gertsch, *The ECG Manual: An Evidence-Based Approach*,
© Springer-Verlag London Limited 2009

ECG 28.1 Electrocardiogram (ECG) obtained from a
49-year-old woman with atrial septal defect of the ostium
secundum type (ASD II), left to right shunt >60%. Pulmonary
artery pressure normal. ECG: frontal QRS axis +105°.
Incomplete right bundle-branch block with r′ > r,
T negative up to lead V_5

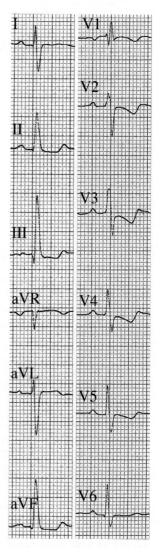

Generally, the pulmonary artery pressure is normal. The regression of ECG
signs of RV hypertrophy/dilatation after operation can last years or remain incomplete. ASD II with small left to right shunt (and of course a patent foramen ovale)
do not result in ECG abnormalities.

Differential Diagnosis of Atrial Septal Defect of the Ostium Secundum Type

1. Abnormal drainage of lung veins (into the right atrium or, rarely, the cava veins)
   with a great left to right shunt show a similar ECG pattern, more often without
   iRBBB.

2. Chronic pulmonary embolism. The diagnosis is made on the basis of anamnestic and clinical findings and echo/Doppler.
3. Acute and subacute pulmonary embolism. In these conditions, the ECG might be similar to that of ASD II. Again, the diagnosis is made on the basis of history, clinical findings, echo/Doppler, d-Dymer, and, if available, helical computed tomography.
4. Valvular pulmonary stenosis. Instead of the great singular R wave in V_1 (in 60%), we find in this lead an rSr' complex (incomplete RSB, in 40%).

Atrial Septal Defect of the Ostium Primum Type (ASD I)

The ECG is characterized by left axis deviation, because of absence or interruption of the left anterior fascicle (ECG 28.2). An iRBBB may or may not be present. Major types of endocardial cushion defects [ASD I + ventricular septal defect and complete atrioventricular (AV) channel] show similar ECGs, occasionally with RBBB, without operation.

Valvular Pulmonary Stenosis

In general, right axis deviation. In approximately 60%, tall R wave in V_1 (ECG 28.3); in approximately 40%, rSr' configuration in V_1 (iRBBB), similar to ASD II. Signs of right atrial enlargement can be present.

Tetralogy of Fallot

Without surgical correction, the ECG is similar to that of valvular pulmonary stenosis (ECG 28.4). After surgical correction, an RBBB pattern is obligatory (ECG 28.5).

Ventricular Septal Defect

A small ventricular septal defect generally does not alter the ECG. Left axis deviation can be present. A great left to right shunt leads to biventricular overload and can show (in children) the "Katz Wachtel sign" (R + S in V_2 or V_3 ≥ 4 mV). Signs of left atrial enlargement can be present.

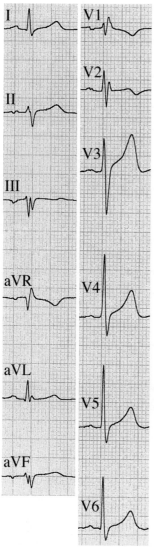

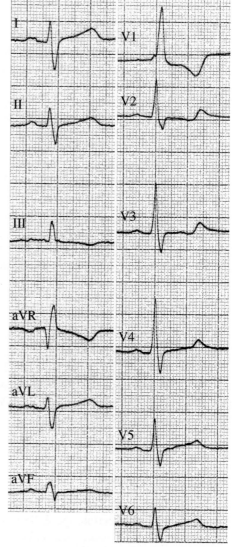

ECG 28.2 Electrocardiogram (ECG) obtained from a 25-year-old man with atrial septal defect of the ostium primum type (ASD I). Left to right shunt 60%. Pulmonary artery pressure minimally increased. ECG: sinus rhythm, left atrial overload (lead V_1: negative portion of the p wave greater than positive portion). Frontal QRS axis –60°. Incomplete right bundle-branch block with r′ > r (lead V_1). T negativity in V_1/V_2

ECG 28.3 Electrocardiogram (ECG) obtained from a 19-year-old man with severe pulmonary valve stenosis (gradient 90 mmHg). ECG (paper speed 50 mm/s): frontal QRS axis +120°. Tall single R wave (15 mm), ST depression, and negative T wave in V_1. R > S in V_2 to V_4. Note that in approximately 40%, the ECGs in pulmonary stenosis show the pattern of incomplete right bundle-branch block, which makes it difficult to distinguish from that of atrial septal defect of the ostium secundum type (ASD II). In ASD II, a single R wave in V_1 is extremely rare

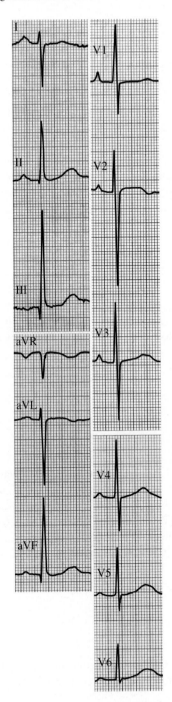

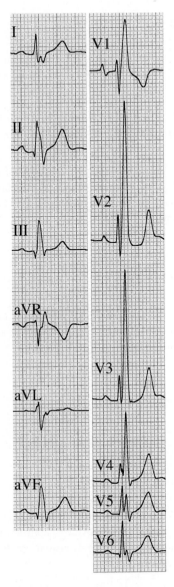

ECG 28.4 Electrocardiogram (ECG) obtained from a 2-year-old boy with Fallot's tetralogy, not operated. ECG (50 mm/s): QRS right axis deviation. R > S in lead V_1, indicating right ventricular hypertrophy

ECG 28.5 Electrocardiogram (ECG) obtained from a 26-year-old man with Fallot's tetralogy operated 10 years previously. ECG: frontal QRS axis (of the first 60 ms) +75°. Direct pattern of right bundle-branch block in V_1 to V_5 (V_6), with giant amplitude of R′ in V_2/V_3, corresponding to persisting severe right ventricular hypertrophy, confirmed by the echo

Patent Ductus Botalli

In babies with great left to right shunt, the rare pattern of left ventricular diastolic overload might be observed. Often, there is left atrial enlargement.

Transposition of the Great Arteries

The $\mathring{A}QRS_F$ depends on the mode of transposition. For all forms, a huge R wave in lead V_1 is common (ECG 28.6). The ECG might be similar to Eisenmenger syndrome. For the ECG of congenitally corrected transposition of the great arteries, see Chapter 14.

Situs Inversus

Situs inversus without additional abnormalities leads to a very typical ECG: Inversion of p and QRS in the limb leads and decrease (instead of increase) of the R voltage in V_4 to V_6 (ECG 28.7).

Ebstein's Anomaly

The so-called typical Ebstein-ECG consists of:

1. Extreme "p pulmonale," with tall p waves in III and AVF and tall/peaky p waves in V_1/V_2
2. Right axis deviation
3. "M" configuration of QRS in leads III and aVF. During 25 years, we have seen this pattern only twice in approximately 30 cases. The ECG alterations are often much more modest, absent, or atypical (ECG 28.8). Even left axis deviation might be present.

Complex Congenital Cardiac Diseases

ECG alterations in complex diseases often show QRS prolongation and signs of RV hypertrophy. However, many other patterns occur, depending on the anomaly.

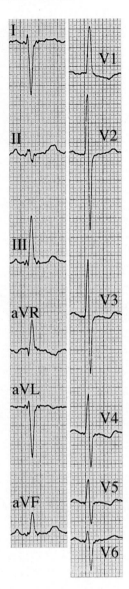

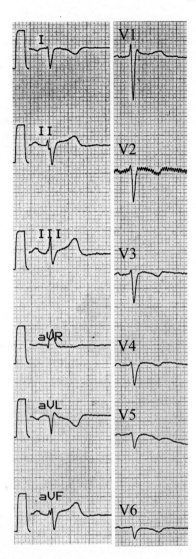

ECG 28.6 Electrocardiogram (ECG) obtained from a 14-year-old girl with d-transposition of the great arteries. Correction by Mustard operation 12 years previously. ECG: sinus rhythm. Frontal QRS axis +160°. Huge R wave in lead V_1 (12 mm). High RS amplitude in V_2/V_3. T negativity in V_1 to V_5

ECG 28.7 Electrocardiogram (ECG) obtained from a 40-year-old man with situs inversus, but otherwise healthy. ECG: typical inversion of p waves and QRS complexes (similar to that in false poling of the upper limb leads). rS complex in all precordial leads, with decreasing r amplitude from V_1 to V_6. ST/T alterations

ECG 28.8 Electrocardiogram (ECG) obtained from a
60-year-old man with Ebstein's anomaly of medium to
severe degree. Right ventricular failure. ECG: sinus
rhythm. Left (!) atrial enlargement. Atrioventricular
block 1°. Frontal QRS axis (first 70 ms) +70°. Complete
right bundle-branch block. T negativity in V_1 to V_3
(to V_6). Note that the ECG does not suggest Ebstein's
anomaly. Left atrial overload, rather than right, is unusual. Also, the so-called "typical M configuration" in
lead III is missed. However, in our experience, these
ECG signs, which should be typical for the disease,
are often missed

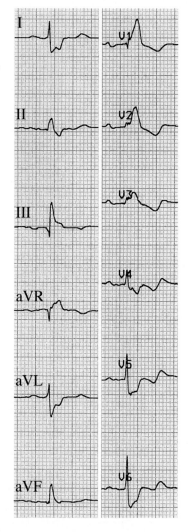

Eisenmenger Syndrome

Eisenmenger reaction, often called Eisenmenger syndrome, can occur in patients
with excessive left to right shunt that leads to alterations of the small pulmonary
artery vessels with consecutive severe ("fixed") pulmonary hypertension. The additional right to left shunt is a consequence of pulmonary hypertension. The ECG is
characterized by often extreme right axis deviation and a tall R wave in V_1 (V_2),
with or without alterations of ST/T in the precordial leads (ECG 28.9).

ECG 28.9 Electrocardiogram (ECG) obtained from a
27-year-old man with huge ventricular septal defect
with early Eisenmenger reaction at the age of 2 years.
ECG: QRS right axis deviation. Single R wave (30 mm)
in V_1. Positive T wave in all precordial leads

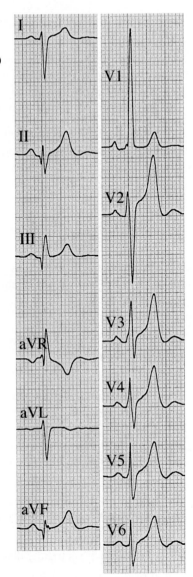

Mitral Valve Prolapse (Barlow's Disease)

Generally, this disease is not connected with a typical ECG. In approximately
5%–10% of cases, negative asymmetric T waves in leads III/aVF and V_6 are
present, a pattern rarely seen in other conditions. In inferolateral ischemia, the
T waves are mostly negative and symmetric.

Hypertrophic Obstructive Cardiomyopathy

Occasionally, the diagnosis is suspected by prominent Q waves in leads I, aVL, and V_4 to V_6 that might be combined with signs of left ventricular hypertrophy (LVH) (see ECGs in Chapters 5 and 14). Following are other possible ECG patterns in hypertrophic obstructive cardiomyopathy:

1. Signs of LVH without prominent Q waves
2. Left bundle-branch block pattern
3. Normal ECG!

Acquired Valvular Heart Diseases

On one hand, the ECG alterations generally depend on the severity of the anomaly, but on the other hand, the ECG might completely fail to show typical alterations, as for instance, LVH.

Valvular Aortic Stenosis

Approximately 60% of these patients show classical signs of LVH, generally with a slightly prolonged QRS and discordant negative asymmetric T waves in leads I, aVL, and V_5/V_6 ("systolic overload"). An $\mathring{A}QRS_F$ between +30° and +60° is not uncommon probably because of concentric LVH. Especially in young adults, the ECG can be normal, even in severe aortic stenosis.

Valvular Aortic Incompetence

The pattern of "left ventricular diastolic overload" is very rarely seen.

1. Tall R waves with deep Q waves in V_4 to V_6, without QRS prolongation
2. Slight ST elevation and tall symmetroid T waves in the same leads

Generally, the ECG pattern cannot be distinguished from that of valvular aortic stenosis (VAS); in advanced aortic incompetence, T inversion in the lateral leads is mostly found. The $\mathring{A}QRS_F$ is generally more to the left than in VAS, between +30° and −10°.

Mitral Stenosis

A pattern of extensive left atrial enlargement ("p mitrale," with a peak-to-peak interval of >40 ms) is found in >60% of cases. In advanced diseases, atrial fibrillation is common. RV hypertrophy is often detectable by a vertical $\mathring{A}QRS_F$ and an iRBBB (ECG 28.10) or a relatively high R wave in V_1.

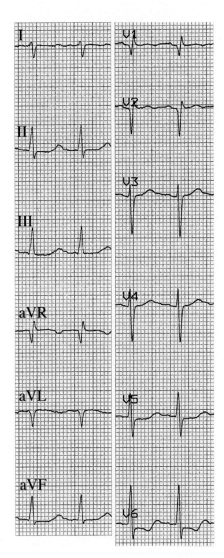

ECG 28.10 Electrocardiogram (ECG) obtained from a 43-year-old woman with severe mitral stenosis with tricuspid regurgitation. Mitral valve replacement and tricuspid De Vega plastic 2 years before. ECG: sinus rhythm 116 beats/min. P duration >200 ms. The first peak of the p wave is partially hidden within the T wave. Atrioventricular block 1°. Frontal QRS axis +115°. Qr in V_1 and V_2. Alteration of the repolarization. Coro: normal

Mitral Incompetence

There are no typical ECG signs. Only in longstanding mitral incompetence, left atrial enlargement (of minor degree than in mitral stenosis) and obvious LVH are found in approximately 30% of cases. Surprisingly, a QRS counterclockwise rotation instead of an expected clockwise rotation, in left ventricular dilatation, might be found.

Chapter 29
Digitalis Intoxication

Digitalis intoxication in its chronic or subacute form occurs mainly in elderly patients with reduced body weight and in patients with renal failure. Based on new data, intoxication is more frequent in women than in men, possibly because of relative overdose. Also, conditions increasing sensibility to digoxin might be important, such as hypothyroidism, hypokalemia and hypomagnesemia, and acute ischemia. Moreover, some drugs, such as quinidine, amiodarone, and spironolactone, increase the serum level of digoxin.

Digitalis intoxication leads to conduction disturbances and arrhythmias. It affects the sinoatrial conduction and the supra-His atrioventricular (AV) conduction system. AV block 1° often develops to AV block 2° of the Wenckebach type and could further progress to AV block 2:1, or, in rare cases, to complete AV block, always with a supra-His escape rhythm and small QRS complexes. In patients with preexisting atrial fibrillation, impaired AV conduction provokes bradycardia. Sinus bradycardia might also be present.

Many arrhythmias result from increased automaticity in the atrium, the AV junction, and the ventricles. The most common arrhythmias are frequent premature beats, especially ventricular premature beats in bigeminy. In severe life-threatening cases, ventricular tachycardia is common. The ventricular tachycardia is often irregular, monomorphic, or polymorphic without torsades de pointes (ECG 29.1) and rarely of the type torsades de pointes. Ventricular fibrillation can occur, as well as cardiac standstill (ECG 29.2). A rare but quite typical arrhythmia, atrial tachycardia with AV block (generally 2:1), is an example of enhanced automaticity and combined conduction impairment (ECG 29.3). It is important to note that digitalis intoxication can provoke nearly all cardiac arrhythmias, even, very rarely, tachycardiac atrial fibrillation. ST depression is seen in patients with normal or pathologic digoxin levels, whereas a striking shortening of the QT interval is observed only in digitalis intoxication.

M. Gertsch, *The ECG Manual: An Evidence-Based Approach,*
© Springer-Verlag London Limited 2009

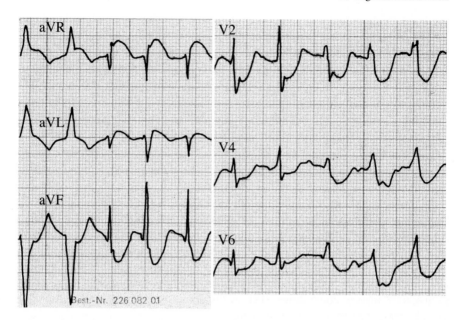

ECG 29.1 Electrocardiogram (ECG) obtained from a 50-year-old woman 4 hours after intake of 30 tablets of digoxin 0.25 mg in a suicide attempt. Serum level 11 nmol/L. ECG (only Goldberger leads, V_2, V_4, V_6; other leads and rhythm strip lost): possible bidirectional ventricular tachycardia. Striking ST depression in some leads

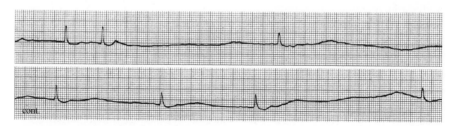

ECG 29.2 Electrocardiogram (ECG) obtained from a 78-year-old woman after subacute overdose of digoxin. Serum level 9.4 nmol/L. ECG (continuous rhythm strip): no p waves detectable. Irregular atrioventricular junctional rhythm with several ventricular pauses up to 3.88 s

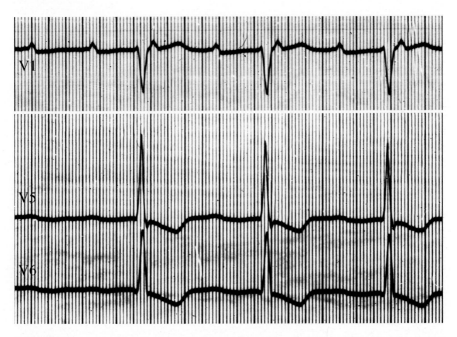

ECG 29.3 Electrocardiogram (ECG) obtained from a 54-year-old man with severe aortic and mitral valve disease. Subacute overdose of digoxin. Serum level 7.2 nmol/L. ECG (paper speed 50 mm/s): atrial tachycardia (atrial rate 170 beats/min) with high-degree atrioventricular block 2°, ventricular rate approximately 85 beats/min

Extracardiac Symptoms

Most of the extracardiac symptoms are as common as nonspecific and include fatigue, weakness, nausea, and vomiting. A combination of these symptoms with visual symptoms such as enhanced perception of yellow and green and seeing halos of light can lead to the correct interpretation. Also, hallucination and delirium have been described.

Severe acute digitalis intoxication represents an extremely dangerous condition and needs a complex emergency treatment. Chronic digitalis intoxication is not a rare situation, because of the still-frequent use of the drug and the mainly nonspecific symptoms. The incidence of toxicity (of various degrees) in digitalized patients varies between 6% and 23%. Most publications deal with digoxin. Based on a recent study, it can be assumed that digoxin increases the mortality in women with heart failure and depressed left ventricular function, in contrast to men. It is believed that this is attributable to a digoxin serum level that is too high in women; therefore, the use of a dose that will result in a serum concentration lower than 1.0 nmol/L in women has been proposed.

Note: The interested reader finds 650 actual *references* in the comprehensive book M. Gertsch, Springer 2004, linked at the end of each of the 32 chapters.

Index

Printed in the United States of America